A PRIMER OF MAGNETIC RESONANCE IMAGING

A PRIMER OF MAGNETIC RESONANCE IMAGING

Jacek W. Hennel

The Niewodniczański Institute of Nuclear Physics
31-342 Kraków, Radzikowskiego 152, Poland

Teresa Kryst-Widźgowska

Institute of Psychiatry and Neurology
Warszawa, Poland

Jacek Klinowski

Department of Chemistry, University of Cambridge
Lensfield Road, Cambridge CB2 1EW, U.K.

Imperial College Press

ICP

Published by

Imperial College Press
203 Electrical Engineering Building
Imperial College
London SW7 2BT

Distributed by

World Scientific Publishing Co. Pte. Ltd.
P O Box 128, Farrer Road, Singapore 912805
USA office: Suite 1B, 1060 Main Street, River Edge, NJ 07661
UK office: 57 Shelton Street, Covent Garden, London WC2H 9HE

British Library Cataloguing-in-Publication Data
A catalogue record for this book is available from the British Library.

ISBN 1-86094-060-9

Printed in Singapore by Uto-Print

PREFACE

This book is concerned with imaging the interior of the human body using signals originating from the magnetic moments of hydrogen nuclei, detected using a technique known as magnetic resonance. We explain how the method works and give examples of its applications.

The book is addressed to those who would like to understand the principle of the method exactly, but do not have university training in physics and mathematics. The book should therefore be useful to inquisitive medical practitioners and researchers, radiologists and auxilliary workers in the health service.

We are grateful to Dr A. Jasinski, Dr P. Sagnowski, Dr F. Hennel and Dr N.A.H. Dawnay for comments on the text, and to Mr P. Kulinowski for preparing the line figures.

The Authors

CONTENTS

Chapter 4. Imaging 41

Chapter 5. Practical Aspects 57

Further Reading 79

Index 83

CHAPTER 1

INTRODUCTION

1.1 Overview

Magnetic Resonance Imaging (MRI) is a powerful method of non-invasive imaging of the interior of a living body for medical diagnostic and other purposes. This is achieved using an instrument known as a tomograph, an example of which is shown in Fig. 1.1. The equipment also contains components not shown in the Figure: the various electronic circuits, a computer and a monitor for displaying the results. MRI must be distinguished from X-ray tomography (CT scanning) which also uses computers for forming images.

The main component of the MRI tomograph shown in Fig. 1.2 is the magnet: an enormous cylindrical coil, which is drawn in a longitudinal cross-section. However, there are imagers with magnets of different construction. The patient, volunteer or other subject is placed inside the coil in its strong and stable magnetic field. Additional coils ("transmitter-receiver coils"), which are part of an electric circuit carrying an alternating current, are located close to the part of the body which is being examined. The current running through the magnet generates a constant magnetic field which interacts with the magnetic moment of protons (nuclei of hydrogen) present in the human body in enormous numbers, especially in water.

The principle of magnetic resonance can be briefly stated in one sentence: certain atomic nuclei (those with the property of "spin") absorb radio waves of a strictly defined frequency when placed in a magnetic field. The basis of the operation of an MRI imager is as follows. When an object containing protons is placed in a strong magnetic field, nuclear magnetization builds up in the entire object. In a homogeneous magnetic field (that of equal strength at any point in space) all individual protons would absorb a pulse of an appropriate radiofrequency. However, when a magnetic field gradient is superimposed on the constant magnetic field,

1

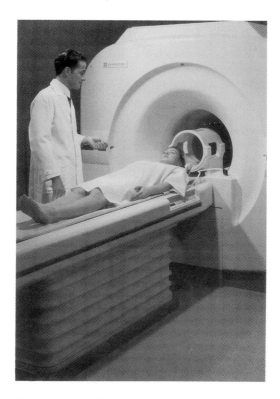

Figure 1.1. Overall view of a Shimatzu MRI tomograph.

the nuclei in each transverse slice of the object experience a different magnetic field. When a radiofrequency field is applied, only the nuclei in a narrow slice will respond to it: the frequency of the pulse is too high for the nuclei experiencing fields smaller than the value B_e in Fig. 1.2, and too low for the nuclei which experience field higher than B_e. In this way, the combination of a field gradient and a radiofrequency pulse selects a slice of the object. By using a pulse of different frequency or a different field gradient, a different slice can be chosen for examination.

An electronic apparatus driven by a computer sends a pulse of alternating current through the transmitter-receiver coils for a fraction of a second, after which the protons stimulated by the current induce in them an electric potential known as the "signal". The frequency of the signal depends on the strength of the constant magnetic field in which the given proton is placed. Only the protons within a thin slice of the object (for example the head, as shown in Fig. 1.2) are excited. Protons from outside the slice are unaffected and do not induce a signal.

The signal from the protons in the slice, composed of superimposed signals from its individual elements, is registered in computer memory. The analysis of the signal from the entire slice is done by the computer using the "Fourier transformation". This provides the information about the intensity of signals from the individual elements of the slice. The image of the slice is simply the intensity map of these signals: the picture of the desired cross-section of the object. Individual organs can be distinguished in the image because different tissues induce the signal differently.

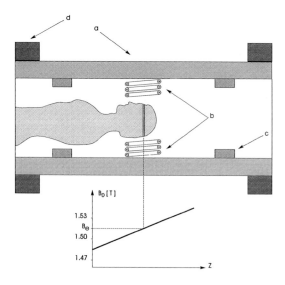

Figure 1.2. Above: Longitudinal cross-section of an MRI tomograph. The coils are shaded. (a) Main coil ("the magnet") generating a strong constant magnetic field; (b) Transmitter-receiver coil which, when connected to a generator of alternating electric current of radio-frequency creates a weak variable magnetic field in the direction perpendicular to that of the constant field; (c) Gradient coils; (d) Shimming coils. An alternating magnetic field generated by the transmitter-receiver coil stimulates magnetic resonance signals in a thin slice of the subject. The computer uses these signals to build an image of the slice. Below: Plot of the intensity of the magnetic field at the centre of the magnet during the application of the magnetic field gradient.

By examining a certain region of the object slice by slice we accumulate and store information about the entire region. Using specially designed software, the computer can then display on the screen cross-sections at any point and any angle. The operator can assess this information even after completing the measurement and sending the patient home.

The same equipment can be used for imaging in many different ways. The various imaging methods are differently suited to specific diagnostic purposes. There is an appropriate computer program for each method, to be chosen according to need. This opens numerous possibilities. We can, for example, adjust the contrast according to various physical properties of the individual tissues, image the cardiovascular system, measure the rate of blood flow and chemically analyse selected regions of the image for the content of specific metabolites. We can also study the functions of the individual parts of the brain.

This book explains the basic principles and the important features of MRI as fully as possible. Our task is not to describe the numerous variations of the technique in detail. Without sacrificing correctness, we have made certain necessary simplifications to enable a reader without advanced knowledge of mathematics and physics to understand the principles of MRI. Chapter 2 summarises the basic necessary mathematical and physical information. Those who are well familiar with mathematics and physics can begin reading from Chapter 3.

CHAPTER 2

THE FUNDAMENTALS

2.1 Periodic Motion

We begin by providing the reader with some information about functions. The term "function" is used to indicate the correspondence between two quantities. The statement $y = f(t)$, read "y is a function of t", indicates the relationship between the variables t (known as the "independent variable") and y (the "dependent variable"). $f(t)$ is usually given as an explicit formula, such as $f(t) = t^2 - 3t + 5$. If a is a number, $f(a)$ is the value of the function for the value $t = a$. Thus in the example given above $f(3) = 3^2 - 3 \times 3 + 5 = 5$ and $f(-4) = 33$. A function can alternatively be specified as a table of the values of $f(t)$ corresponding to various values of the variable t.

Consider a point R lying on the circumference of a circle of radius r, and two mutually perpendicular axes crossing at the centre (Fig. 2.1). The axes form the so-called "coordinate system". The distances of point R from the axes are the coordinates: the coordinate x, equal to the length OG is the distance from the Y axis, and the coordinate y, equal to the length OF, is the distance from the X axis. The position of a point is unambiguously determined by its coordinates. The points G and F are the "projections" of the point R onto the respective axes.

The coordinates x and y of the point R are related to the angle the radius OR makes with the axis X via the trigonometric functions $\sin \alpha$ and $\cos \alpha$

$$\sin \alpha = \frac{y}{r} \qquad\qquad \cos \alpha = \frac{x}{r} \;.$$

By multiplying both sides of the above equations by r we find the coordinates in terms of the angle α

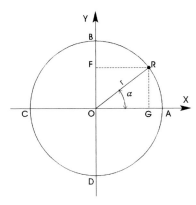

Figure 2.1. Point R lying on the circumference of a circle of radius r. When the point moves with a constant velocity along the circumference, the angle α changes as $\alpha = \omega t$, where ω is the angular velocity. The angle α, known as the phase, determines the position of point R at time t. If the motion began when point R was at position A, the angle α may be considered as the angular path traversed during time t. The x coordinate of point R is a function of time: $x(t) = r \cos \omega t$. The plot of this function is a cosine curve.

$$x = r \cos \alpha \qquad (2.1)$$

$$y = r \sin \alpha . \qquad (2.2)$$

Imagine that the point R moves with a constant velocity in the counter-clockwise sense along the circumference of the circle. Such motion is equivalent to the rotation of the radius OR. At time $t = 0$ the point R lies on the X axis and coincides with point A; after time t it finds itself at the position shown in Fig. 2.1. The total angle may be considered as the path traversed by OR during time t. Since path = velocity × time, we can write

$$\alpha = \omega t \qquad (2.3)$$

where ω is known as the angular velocity. The angle which determines the position of radius OR at time t is known as the phase. Substituting

Eq. (2.3) into Eq. (2.1) and Eq (2.2) we obtain the coordinates of point R a t any instant during the course of the motion, i.e. as a function of time:

$$x(t) = r \cos \omega t$$

$$y(t) = r \sin \omega t .$$

Fig. 2.2 shows the plots of the function r cos ωt.

When measured in units of radians per second (2π radians correspond to one full revolution of 360 degrees, so that 1 radian = 57.296 degrees), angular velocity is denoted by ω, and when measured in numbers of full revolutions per second, by v. We shall refer to both quantities as "frequency", because they differ only by a constant coefficient:

$$\omega = 2\pi \, v .$$

The "period" T is the time needed for one full revolution. We have therefore

$$v = \frac{1}{T} \quad \text{and} \quad \omega = \frac{2\pi}{T} .$$

The unit of frequency is one period per second, known as 1 hertz (Hz). A million hertz is a megahertz (MHz).

It is clear from Fig. 2.1 that the values of the function cos α are all found in the interval from –1 to +1. Thus when the moving point R coincides with A, $x(t) = r$ and cos $\omega t = 1$; when it coincides with C then $x(t) = -r$ and cos $\omega t = -1$.

Many physical processes proceed according to the relationship A cos ωt, where A is a constant. One example is the oscillation of a weight suspended from a spring. After lifting the weight and letting it go at the height $h = A$ from the position of equilibrium, the weight oscillates about the equilibrium position. The distance from equilibrium is a function of time:

$$h(t) = A \cos \omega t .$$

The time needed for the weight to return to position A is the period T, while the constant A, corresponding to the maximum deflection is known as the amplitude.

Another example of a change proceeding according to the A cos ωt relationship is the alternating electric current which varies from a certain maximum value A to a minimum at –A (when it flows in the opposite direction). In European countries there are 50 full A → –A → A cycles per second, so that v = 50 Hz and ω = 314.159 radians per second. In the U.S.A. v = 60 Hz and ω = 376.991 radians per second. These examples show that ω and v are not only useful when dealing with *actual* rotation.

In radio circuits the current and the voltage change much faster than in the electric grid. For example, the range of short waves spans the frequencies from 1.6 to 22 MHz, and the range of very short waves (VHF) runs from 67 to 108 MHz. MRI uses frequencies from tens to hundreds of MHz.

It often happens that physical changes (mechanical, electrical, magnetic etc.) cannot be described by a single function A cos ωt, but by a sum of such functions, each with a different frequency and amplitude (Fig. 2.2a–2.2c). Fig. 2.2d shows the plot of such a composite function. The question arises of how to determine the composition of a curve with a known shape or, in other words, how to decompose it into individual cosine curves. This question is fundamental to MRI, because the formation of the image is based on such decomposition. The answer is a mathematical procedure known as the Fourier transformation.

Before we explain the Fourier transformation, we must give the reader some facts about integration. The integral of an arbitrary function $f(t)$ is the area between the plot of the function and the axis of the variable t starting from some value $t = A$ to some other value $t = B$. However, we count the area above the axis as positive and the area below the axis as negative (Fig. 2.3a). The integral is therefore an algebraic sum of the areas above and below the x axis within the specified limits.

The integral of the function cos ωt over a full period, i.e. for B – A = T, is zero (Fig. 2.4a), because the areas above and below the axis are equal and cancel one another. This result is independent of the choice of the lower limit of integration A. The important consequence of this is that, when we integrate a larger section of cos ωt, full periods do not contribute to the integral, and only any incomplete period needs to be taken into account (Fig. 2.4b).

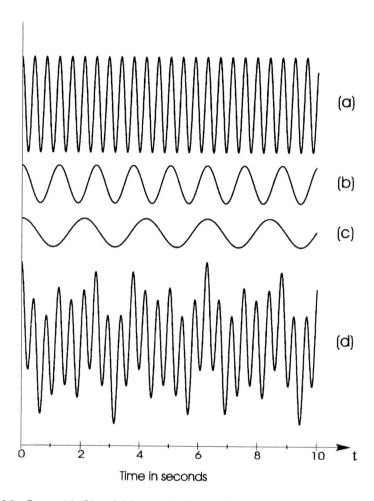

Time in seconds

Figure 2.2. Curves (a), (b) and (c) are individual cosine curves, i.e. plots of the function $f(t) = A \cos \omega t$ for different values of frequency ω and amplitude A: (a) $\omega = 15$, A = 5; (b) $\omega = 5$, A = 2; (c) $\omega = 3$, A = 1.5. Curve (d) is the sum of these three cosine curves, i.e. the plot of the function $f(t) = 5 \cos 15t + 2 \cos 5t + 1.5 \cos 3t$. This function cannot be decomposed into the individual cosine functions by visual examination. Analysis of complicated curves requires the Fourier transformation.

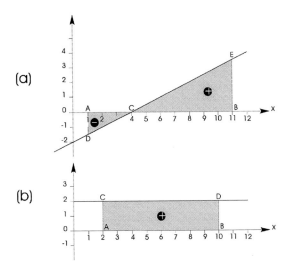

Figure 2.3. Examples of integration. (a) Integral of the function $f(t) = 0.5\, x - 2$ (the plot of which is the straight line DE) between the limits $A = 1$ and $B = 11$ is equal to the sum of the areas of triangles DAC with a negative sign and CEB with a positive sign. Applying the formula for the area of a right-angled triangle we obtain the value of the integral as $0.5 \times (1.5 \times -3 + 7 \times 3.5) = 10$. (b) Integral of the constant function $f(x) = 2$ between the limits from 2 to 10 is equal to the area of the rectangle ACDB with a positive sign, i.e. $2 \times 8 = 16$.

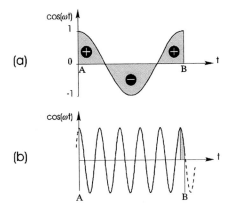

Figure 2.4. (a) Section of the curve cos ωt corresponding to one full revolution of point R, i.e. to one full period. The integral of the interval is zero: the areas above and below the time axis are identical and, having opposite signs, cancel one another. Integration shown above begins at $A = 0$, but the integral is always zero whatever the lower limit of integration, as long as $B - A = T$. (b) Integral within a longer time interval, involving a larger number of periods, is equal only to the integral of the last incomplete period (shaded), because full periods do not contribute.

2.2 A Few Words About Vectors

We often encounter physical quantities which have not only magnitude (expressed numerically in the appropriate units) but also direction. Such quantities are known as vectors. A well known example of a vector is force. In order to describe a force it is not sufficient to give its magnitude in the appropriate units: the direction must also be given. In this book we shall come across the vectors of the magnetic field, magnetic field gradient and magnetic moment.

Vectors are graphically represented by arrows, with the direction of the arrow giving the direction of the vector and the length describing its magnitude. Vectors are usually written in bold type, and their magnitude in ordinary type. For example, the magnitude of a vector **F** is written as F.

Vectors are added just as forces: using the parallelogram rule (Fig. 2.5a). A sum of vectors is known as the resultant vector. The parallelogram rule can also be applied to decompose a vector into a sum of two vectors pointing in the required directions. For example, we often need to decompose a vector into components in the directions of the X and Y axes of the coordinate system. Since the axes are mutually perpendicular, the parallelogram is then a rectangle (Fig. 2.5b). A three-dimensional coordinate system has three mutually perpendicular axes: X, Y and Z. The spatial decomposition of a vector into components will be discussed in Section 2.4 on p. 16.

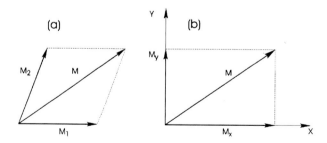

Figure 2.5. (a) Addition of vectors. The vector sum **M** is the diagonal of the parallelogram formed by vectors **M₁** and **M₂** which are being added. (b) Decomposition of vector **M** into components **Mₓ** and **Mᵧ** lying along the X and Y axes of the coordinate system.

2.3 The Fourier Transformation

We saw in Section 2.1 that the sum of several cosine curves is a complicated curve $f(t)$ (Fig. 2.2d). We shall now consider the reverse problem which can be stated as follows:

1. Can an arbitrary function $f(t)$ be represented by a sum of cosines?
2. If so, how is one to find the frequencies and amplitudes of the component cosine functions?

The answer to the first question is yes (with certain exceptions which are unimportant here) and is given by the Fourier Theorem. The theorem, which we use without proof, states that any function $f(t)$, specified either as a plot or as a list of numbers, is equivalent to a sum of cosine functions:

$$f(t) = F(\omega_1) \cos \omega_1 t + F(\omega_2) \cos \omega_2 t + \ldots \qquad (2.4)$$

and that the amplitudes $F(\omega_1)$, $F(\omega_2)$, ... can always be calculated. The values $F(\omega_1)$, $F(\omega_2)$, ... are treated here as numbers. Later, the set of these numbers will be treated as a function of frequency, $F(\omega)$.

The answer to the second question is the so-called Fourier transformation, a mathematical procedure leading to the amplitudes $F(\omega)$. In simple terms, this procedure consists of converting a function of time $f(t)$ into a function of frequency $F(\omega)$. In principle, the Fourier transformation answers the question only for an arbitrarily chosen frequency ω_x, by telling us whether $\cos \omega_x t$ appears in Eq. (2.4), and if so with what amplitude. In order to pick out all the frequencies which appear in this sum, the transformation has to be carried out repeatedly, each time with a different value of ω_x.

The Fourier transformation consists of two steps. We first multiply the function we wish to transform by $\cos \omega_x t$, and then integrate the result within very wide limits of t (the concept of integration has been outlined in Section 2.1). We need therefore to integrate the product

$$f(t) \cos \omega_x t \, .$$

The task is simplified by writing the function $f(t)$ in the form of Eq. (2.4), giving

$$f(t) \cos \omega_x t = F(\omega_1) \cos \omega_1 t \cos \omega_x t + F(\omega_2) \cos \omega_2 t \cos \omega_x t + \dots .(2.5)$$

An integral of a sum is equal to the sum of integrals of the individual terms. We therefore integrate each of the terms in Eq. (2.5) separately and add the results. We first transform Eq. (2.5) using the formula for the product of two cosines from basic trigonometry

$$\cos \alpha \cos \beta = \frac{1}{2} \left[\cos (\alpha + \beta) + \cos (\alpha - \beta) \right] .$$

In this way we have

$$F(\omega_i) \cos \omega_i t \cos \omega_x t = \frac{1}{2} F(\omega_i) \left[\cos(\omega_i + \omega_x)t + \cos (\omega_i - \omega_x)t \right] + \dots (2.5a)$$

We now "try" a particular value of ω_x. There are two distinct possibilities.

(i) Our guess was wrong and the frequency ω_x is different from ω_1, ω_2 etc. All terms on the right-hand-side of Eq. (2.5a) are then cosines with frequencies $\omega_x + \omega_1$, $\omega_x + \omega_2$ etc. and $\omega_x - \omega_1$, $\omega_x - \omega_2$ etc. However, we know from Section 2.1 (Fig. 2.4b), that the integral of a large stretch of a cosine is practically zero. It follows that the value of the whole integral Eq. (2.5a) will be zero as well.

(ii) Our guess was correct and the frequency ω_x coincides with one of the frequencies on the right-hand-side of Eq. (2.5a), say with $\omega_i = \omega_1$. When $\omega_x = \omega_1$, the second term in the square brackets in Eq. (2.5a) is no longer a cosine but a constant, since $\cos (\omega_x - \omega_1) t = \cos 0 = 1$, and we know that the integral of a non-zero constant function is non-zero. The integral of the first term in the square brackets in Eq (2.5a), containing $\cos (\omega_1 + \omega_x)$, is zero, just as for $\omega_x \neq \omega_1$. So are the integrals of expressions in all other square brackets, because $\omega_x \neq \omega_2$, $\omega_x \neq \omega_3$ etc. It follows that when $\omega_x = \omega_1$ the value of the entire integral in Eq. (2.5a) is $\frac{1}{2} F(\omega_1) (t_2 - t_1)$, where $(t_2 - t_1)$ is the length of the integration interval (Fig. 2.3b). Introducing $k = \frac{1}{2}(t_2 - t_1)$ we can rewrite the result of the integration in the form

$$k \, F(\omega_1) . \tag{2.6}$$

Note that in order for Eq. (2.6) to be non-zero, it is not necessary that the condition $\omega_x = \omega_1$ be met exactly. For α close to zero the value of $\cos\alpha$ is very close to unity, so that the Eq (2.6) is also obtained when the values of ω_1 and ω_x are slightly different as long as the product $(\omega_1 - \omega_x)\,t$ is close to zero in the entire interval from t_1 to t_2. This "limited tolerance" allows us to find all the terms in Eq. (2.4).

In practice we know the interval in which all the component frequencies ω_x are to be found. If we examine this interval using densely spaced trial values of ω_x, we shall discover all the components together with their amplitudes. In other words, we shall obtain the relationship between the frequency ω and the amplitude $F(\omega)$ with which this frequency appears in the function $f(t)$. The function $F(\omega)$ is known as the Fourier transform of function $f(t)$. In MRI the function $f(t)$ represents the result of a measurement and the Fourier transform $F(\omega)$ gives the brightness of the individual elements of the image.

The constant k is the same for all ω_1, ω_2 etc. Since, in order to construct the image, we only need the *relative* brightness of the elements, we can divide all the results by k and disregard this constant in further arguments.

2.4 Magnetic Moments and Magnetic Fields

We now consider the concept of a magnetic moment. Given freedom of movement, a body endowed with a magnetic moment always aligns itself in the magnetic field in the same way. The presence of a magnetic moment involves north (N) and south (S) magnetic poles and the generation of a magnetic field. The magnetic moment is a vector which can be imagined as an arrow fixed to a magnetized body which, after the body has aligned itself in the field, points from S to N.

A compass needle is a well-known example of a body with a magnetic moment (Fig. 2.6a). The magnetic moment of the needle comes from the permanent magnetization of the hard steel of which it is made. Electric currents are also accompanied by magnetic effects. Consider a coil made of copper wire which cannot be permanently magnetized. However, when a current flows through the coil, the coil acquires a magnetic moment and a magnetic field appears in and around it (Fig. 2.6b). So, any object with a magnetic moment acts as a magnet generating a magnetic field. The lines of field are closed curves (Fig. 2.6b): outside the magnet they run from the north pole to the south; inside, the other way round.

The vector of the magnetic field may have different magnitudes and directions at different points. The direction of the field at a given point is indicated by the field lines passing through this point. The magnitude of the field, usually given in units of 1 tesla (1 T), may depend on a number of factors.

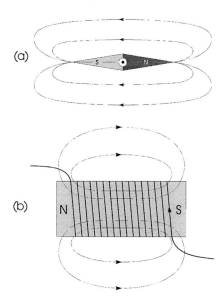

Figure 2.6. Lines of the magnetic field of (a) compass needle; (b) coil. The field is most homogeneous at the centre of the coil, where the lines are parallel to one another. The direction of the magnetic field at any given point is always at a tangent to the line of field passing through that point.

The strength of the field inside a coil depends on the current flowing through the wire and decreases near the ends of the coil. Its direction is parallel to the axis of the coil, apart from small regions close to its ends. A very long and densely wound coil generates a homogeneous field in its interior: a field which has constant magnitude and direction. In reality, however, we use coils of limited length. As a result, the lines of the field diverge and its magnitude decreases towards each end (Fig. 2.6b). This effect is independent of whether the the coil is wound with one or more layers of wire. The size of the region of optimum homogeneity can be increased by placing near the ends of the coil additional correction coils which partially compensate for the decreased field strength (Fig. 2.8b).

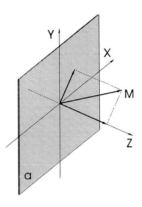

Figure 2.7. Decomposition of vector **M** into the longitudinal component M_z and the transverse component $M_\perp$. The letter "a" marks the transverse plane. It is customary to fix the Z axis in such a way that it coincides with the direction of the magnetic field B_0.

An MRI imager contains several coils. The largest, known as "the magnet", generates a strong and constant magnetic field B_0. The patient is inserted into the magnet in a supine position on a special stretcher. The strength of the main field varies for different imagers from 0.1 to 3 T. The field B_0 should not be confused with the much weaker variable magnetic field generated by the additional coils marked by "b" in Fig. 1.2.

The direction of the magnetic field B_0 is particularly important and is known as the "longitudinal direction". This is conventionally taken to coincide with the direction of the Z axis of the three-dimensional coordinate system. The other two axes, X and Y, are perpendicular to B_0 and determine a plane known as the "transverse plane". In such a coordinate system any vector **M** (Fig. 2.7) can be decomposed into a component in the direction of the Z axis (the longitudinal component M_z) and a component in the transverse plane (the transverse component $M_\perp$). Whenever required, the latter may be further decomposed into components in the X and Y directions.

Using another pair of additional coils, in which the currents flow in opposite directions, we can increase the magnitude of the field gradually, for example from left to right (Fig. 2.8c). By doing this we impose a "field gradient" in the direction of the axis of the coil, i.e. apply a G_z gradient. Using other gradient coils (not shown in Fig. 2.8) we can impose similar gradients (G_x and G_y gradients) along the X and Y axes. As we shall see, gradients are essential for the generation of the image. Gradient coils must be constructed in such a way as not to obstruct the patient, and the variation of the field must be linear. This condition, necessary for the fidelity of the image, is easiest to achieve when the main magnetic field is homogeneous.

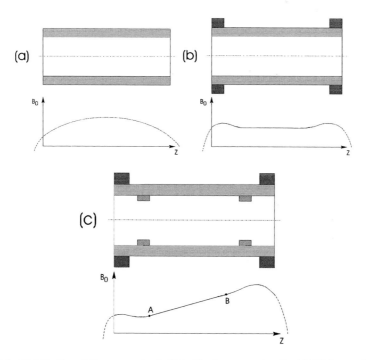

Figure 2.8. Distribution of the magnetic field inside the magnet coil. (a) Without additional coils; (b) With correction coils alone; (c) With correction coils and gradient coils. Gradient coils are connected to the current source in opposite senses. In the region from A to B the magnetic field B_0 increases linearly along the Z axis, which is known as the G_z gradient. Gradients G_x and G_y along the X and Y axes are obtained using coils of different shape and configuration (not shown).

The rest of this section is concerned with the construction of magnets. Knowledge of this is not necessary for understanding the principles of MRI and the section can therefore be omitted at first reading.

MRI uses two kinds of magnets: superconducting magnets (without a core) (Figs. 1.2 and 2.8) and iron-core electromagnets. Superconducting magnets, with coils made of superconducting wire kept at a very low temperature in a liquid helium bath, are now the most common. The axis of the magnet is horizontal, which enables easy manipulation of the patient in the supine position.

Superconductivity was discovered in 1911 by the Dutch scientist H. Kamerlingh Onnes, who found that some metals, when cooled in liquid helium to the temperature of 4.2 degrees Kelvin (–269°C) completely lose their electrical resistance. Such metals are known as superconductors. A current injected into a superconductor continues to flow even when the source of voltage is disconnected. Certain metallic alloys which superconduct even in the presence of very high magnetic fields are suitable for the construction of superconducting magnets. An alloy of titanium-niobium is now commonly used. The "wire" is in fact a braid of many very thin wires made of the superconducting alloy and pressed into a copper wire. The copper protects the superconductor and ensures thermal contact with the liquid helium, but does not carry any current. As a non-superconductor, copper forces the current, which always chooses the path of least resistance, to flow through the thin alloy braid. While in a superconducting state, the hair-like wires can carry very large currents, so that the total current may be as large as 100 amperes. If such a current were to flow through the protective copper lining, it would melt it in an instant. The flow of very large currents through the superconducting braid enables such magnets to generate very large fields.

A superconducting coil immersed in a liquid helium bath has zero electrical resistance. Once injected into it, the current does not decay, so that the coil may be disconnected from the source of potential. This decreases the flow of heat to the liquid helium thus reducing the rate of evaporation. The current is very stable and changes by no more than 0.00001% per hour. Energizing the magnet once is sufficient for many years' work provided that the liquid helium reservoir is regularly replenished. The level of helium must not drop below the top of the coil. Were the coil to emerge from the liquid, a so-called "quench" would inevitably occur:

this is a rapid loss of superconductivity followed by the generation of resistive heat and instantaneous evaporation of the remaining helium.

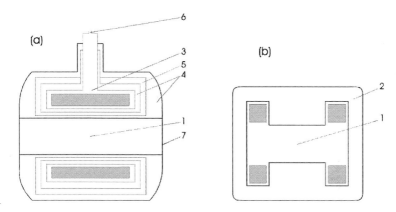

Figure 2.9. Cross-section of two different magnets used in MRI. The coils are shaded. (a) Superconducting magnet with a cryostat; (b) Electromagnet. Legend: 1 – region of maximum field homogeneity in which the imaged object is placed. 2 – iron core. 3 – liquid helium vessel in which the superconducting coil is immersed. 4 – vacuum shield. 5 – liquid nitrogen vessel. 6 – inlet for adding liquid helium and letting off the helium gas. 7 – evacuated outer vessel.

The coil is placed inside a special device known as a cryostat. Its function is to keep the coil in the liquid helium and isolate it from sources of heat while still making it possible for the operator to access the magnetic field at room temperature. The cryostat (Fig. 2.9a) consists of three metal containers placed one inside another like a Russian doll. The innermost container holds the coil and the liquid helium. The second container has double walls with liquid nitrogen in between and protects the helium container from thermal radiation (the boiling point of liquid nitrogen is -196°C). The outermost container is an evacuated shield. The helium and nitrogen vessels are suspended within the vacuum container on thin-walled tubes of stainless steel, which have very poor thermal conductivity. Apart from this, the vessels do not touch one another, and the space between them is kept under high vacuum, which ensures good thermal insulation. The principle is the same as that of a vacuum flask.

Each container is built rather like a doughnut, with a tube passing through its centre and the centre of the coil, so that the patient and all ancillary equipment working in the magnetic field are at room temperature. In modern cryostats the liquid helium bath is extremely well insulated and does not need replenishing more often than once every few months. However, liquid nitrogen, considerably cheaper than liquid helium, needs to be supplied more frequently.

The principal advantage of superconducting magnets is that they generate very strong and very homogeneous fields. At present, 0.5 T, 1.5 T, 2 T and 3 T magnets with bore diameters up to 1 m are commercially available. A superconducting magnet does not require a power supply and thus does not consume energy. The only cost is that of the liquid helium and nitrogen. The drawback of superconducting magnets is their high initial cost. A different problem, but also cost-related, are the strong and extensive stray magnetic fields which easily penetrate walls of buildings and can stop a heart pacemaker even at a distance of several metres. Coming near the magnet with a steel item in one's pocket may result in the item being "sucked" into the bore of the magnet. This may be very dangerous to any patient who happens to be inside, while the collision with the walls of the magnet can cause extensive mechanical damage, or even a quench. Superconducting magnets must therefore be carefully protected from unauthorized personnel, even at a distance of several metres. This applies even to the neighbouring rooms. MRI imagers with superconducting magnets are normally located in fenced purpose-built buildings. The extent of the stray field can be considerably reduced by using shields made of thick iron elements or by additional superconducting coils. However, such installations are very expensive.

Electromagnets are sometimes used in MRI for generating the main magnetic field. The most common design of an electromagnet is schematically shown in Fig. 2.9b. An ordinary (non-superconducting) copper wire is wound onto an iron core. The closed lines of the magnetic field are mostly contained inside an iron yoke, but must traverse the narrow free space known as the gap. The current passing through the coil of an electromagnet is only needed for magnetizing the iron – the real source of the field. However, electromagnets cannot generate very strong magnetic fields because of the so-called "magnetic saturation" of iron. It is also more difficult to make the field homogeneous within a large volume. Electromagnets used in MRI usually work at fields below ca. 0.3 T. The drawback of electromagnets is that they consume large amounts of energy which is given off in the coil as heat, so that the cost of the electricity and of cooling the coil must both be taken into account. On the other hand, electromagnets are cheaper to buy than superconducting magnets and generate much smaller stray fields.

The initial cost and the running costs as well as the range of applications of an imager therefore depend on whether a superconducting magnet or an electromagnet is chosen. The use of magnetic fields of different strengths in different aspects of MRI will be discussed in Section 4.3.

2.5 Electromagnetic Induction

In Section 2.4 we discussed the generation of magnetic fields by electric currents. We shall now consider the reverse effect, in which magnetic field generates electric voltage and electric current.

The principle is as follows. Voltage is induced in a conductor placed in a magnetic field when the field varies in such a way that the changing lines of field cross the conductor. For example, when a magnetic needle is rotated inside a wire coil, the lines of field of the needle criss-cross the turns of the coil. A measuring instrument connected to the coil will detect potential and an alternating current will flow through the entire circuit. The frequency of this current will be equal to the frequency with which the needle is rotated. Generation of voltage and current by a variable magnetic field, known as electromagnetic induction, was discovered by the British physicist Michael Faraday. It is the principle of action of electric generators and also plays an important role in MRI.

2.6 Sampling the Potential

The basis of the generation of an MRI image is the potential induced by magnetic moments contained in the object which is being examined. This potential, which changes with time and can be expressed as a function $f(t)$, is known as the "signal". The signal, which is analogous to a radio or televison signal received by an antenna, carries the desired information and must be measured and sent to the computer for mathematical treatment, in order to determine the brightness of the individual elements of the image.

Computer memory can receive the function $f(t)$ only as a series of numbers. We must therefore represent it as a table in which the values of t are assigned to the corresponding values of $f(t)$. We thus have a finite numer of pairs of numbers describing measurements made at equal time intervals. All this is done by an automatic electronic device known as the analogue-to-digital converter (ADC) which measures the voltage $f(t)$ at time intervals Δt (Fig. 2.10). The result of each measurement is a number expressed in arbitrary, but known units. The string of numbers is then sent to computer memory in the appropriate order, so as not to create confusion as to which value of time t each value of $f(t)$ belongs. In other words, the function $f(t)$ enters the computer memory in a tabular form. This method of converting a continuous function $f(t)$ into a table of numbers by making measurements at equal time intervals is known as "sampling". With modern electronic devices the duration of each actual sampling is so short as to be negligible. Only the sampling interval Δt is important.

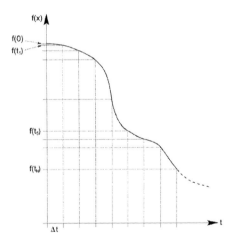

Figure 2.10. Sampling of the MRI signal. A time-dependent voltage $f(t)$ is measured at equal time intervals Δt. The series of results $f(0)$, $f(t_1)$, ... , $f(t_N)$ is equivalent to a continuous function $f(t)$ as long as the spacing between the successive measurements is sufficiently small.

It might appear at first glance that sampling does not give the computer full information about the function, because it does not tell the computer about what happens to $f(t)$ between the sampled values.

Fortunately, information theory tells us that as long as $f(t)$ changes gradually (without sudden jumps) there is always a value of Δt for which the table, albeit discontinuous, contains full information about the function. This means that the missing intermediate values of $f(t)$ can be calculated from the values already in the table. In other words, for a certain value of Δt the function is sampled sufficiently densely, and increased sampling density does not increase the information content of the table. In our further arguments we tacitly assume that sampling is always sufficiently dense.

2.7 Atomic Nuclei

MRI is based on certain properties of atomic nuclei present in the object under study. The nucleus of an atom consists of protons, which carry the elementary positive electric charge, and neutrons which are uncharged. The total nuclear charge depends therefore on the number of constituent protons, and is known as the atomic number Z. Since the atom as a whole must be electrically neutral, the positive charge of the nucleus must be balanced by the negative charge of the electrons. The electric charges of the proton and the electron are equal in magnitude but have opposite signs. It follows that the number of electrons surrounding the nucleus must be equal to the number of protons. In turn, the chemical properties of an atom depend on the number of electrons, and the number Z decides to which element a given atom belongs. It also determines the position of a given element in the Periodic Table.

The mass number A is another important nuclear property. This is the total number of particles in the nucleus, i.e. the sum of the number of neutrons and protons. As the masses of the proton and the neutron are equal, the number A determines the total mass of the nucleus.

Since the atomic number Z alone decides the identity of an atom, it is possible to have nuclei of a given element with different values of A, i.e. with a different number of neutrons. These variants are known as isotopes of a given element, and are distinguished by writing the mass number as a superscript on the left of the symbol of the element. For example, hydrogen has two naturally occurring isotopes: ordinary hydrogen ^{1}H which is 99.98% abundant, and deuterium ^{2}H with a much lower abundance of 0.02%. The nucleus of ordinary hydrogen is simply a single proton, while the nucleus of deuterium contains one proton and one neutron. Oxygen has $Z = 16$ and is a mixture of three isotopes: ^{16}O (99.76%), ^{17}O (0.04%) and ^{18}O (0.2%). There are also elements with only one naturally occurring isotope, such as fluorine ^{19}F and phosphorus ^{31}P.

Although they have the same atomic number Z, isotopes of a given element may differ considerably in many respects. Their suitability for MRI may also be very different. So far, protons, the nuclei of hydrogen, have the greatest, not to say exclusive, application in MRI. They give the strongest nuclear magnetic resonance signal of all isotopes of all elements and are very abundant in living organisms. Protons are present in fats, proteins and above all else in water, which accounts for more than 60% of human body weight. Phosphorus ^{31}P is found in living creatures in much lower quantities, but still gives a measurable resonance signal. At present, phosphorus is not used for imaging, but is important to localized spectroscopy (see Section 4.6).

Apart from the stable isotopes discussed above, there are also unstable radioactive isotopes. These undergo spontaneous nuclear reactions which may generate ionizing radiation dangerous to life. In general, radioactive isotopes are made artificially in nuclear reactors and particle accelerators. **It is important to stress that MRI relies entirely on non-radioactive natural isotopes which are normally found in living matter. It does not use ionizing radiation.**

CHAPTER 3

MAGNETIC BEHAVIOUR OF THE NUCLEUS

3.1 Nuclear Magnetization

Many atomic nuclei undergo very fast rotation, which results in the property known as spin, characteristic of each kind of nucleus. The nucleus carries a positive electric charge, and a rotating charge generates a magnetic field, just as does an electric current running in a closed loop. Nuclei with zero spin, such as those of ^{16}O, the main isotope of oxygen, do not have a magnetic moment. The proton, the nucleus of hydrogen, has the largest magnetic moment of all naturally occurring nuclei.

The behaviour of nuclear magnetic moments immersed in a magnetic field is a matter of fundamental importance. It is quite different from the behaviour of macroscopic objects endowed with magnetic moments, because sub-microscopic entities such as atomic nuclei obey the laws of quantum mechanics. As a result, the nucleus can align its magnetic moment not only in the direction of the field, as a compass needle does, but also in the opposite sense.

When a sample containing atomic nuclei with non-zero spin (such as protons) is immersed in a magnetic field, at first precisely half of the nuclear magnetic moments align with the field and the other half align in the opposite sense. The magnetic moments of the nuclei cancel and do not give rise to an overall moment. However, after a certain period a small portion of the nuclei, so far aligned against the field, reverse their orientation, so that there is a very small surplus of nuclei aligned with the field. This redistribution of orientations of nuclear spins, known as "longitudinal relaxation", does not lead to all magnetic moments aligning themselves in the same direction, because two opposing processes are at work. On the one hand, the field tries to align all spins with itself; on the other, random thermal motions of molecules disorder the spins. A state is finally reached, known as "thermal equilibrium", in which the overall degree of ordering does not change any longer. The stronger the magnetic field and the lower the temperature, the higher the degree of ordering a t thermal equilibrium. However, under normal conditions the degree of ordering is always very small. At room temperature, even in the strongest magnetic fields used for MRI only about five more protons are aligned with the field than against the field per every million protons.

However, this exceedingly small degree of ordering of nuclear magnetic moments is extremely important. Consider the protons of water, which accounts for ca. 60% of human body weight. Since $1 \, cm^3$ of water contains ca. 7×10^{22} protons, the excess number of protons with magnetic moments aligned with the field is ca. $7 \times 10^{22} \times 5/10^6 = 3.5 \times 10^{17}$. This is an enormous number, and the total magnetic moment of these excess protons, known as *nuclear magnetization,* can induce measurable resonance signals and give rise to an MRI image.

3.2 Longitudinal Relaxation

Magnetization created in the process of longitudinal relaxation (Section 3.1) is directed exclusively along the Z axis (so that it has the "longitudinal" direction). As equilibrium is approached, the magnetization grows towards a certain limiting value. We denote this value by M_∞ because, strictly speaking, one would have to wait infinitely long for it to be reached (Fig. 3.1). Relaxation is thus an "exponential process", the characteristic feature of which is that during equal periods of time the value of the magnetization changes by the same fraction of the distance separating it from the limiting value M_∞. This exponential approach to M_∞ is described by the constant T_1, known as the longitudinal relaxation time: the time required to reduce the distance from the target value of M_∞ to 1/3 of the initial distance (strictly speaking to $1/e$, where $e = 2.71828...$ is the base of natural logarithms). Thus after $2T_1$ the distance from M_∞ is reduced to 1/3 of 1/3 (i.e. to 1/9), after $3T_1$ to 1/27, after $4T_1$ to 1/81 etc. After $4T_1$ the remaining distance is so small (1.83%) that we can neglect it and assume that M_∞ has been reached. The error caused by this assumption is insignificant in comparison with the limited accuracy with which the magnetization is measured.

The relaxation time T_1 of protons depends on the substance and in human tissues varies between 200 and 500 milliseconds (1 millisecond, abbreviated as 1 ms is equal to 1/1000 of a second). In very pure water, free of dissolved oxygen, T_1 of protons at 20°C is 3100 milliseconds (3.1 seconds). Dissolved oxygen from the air shortens this value to 2.7 s. Other paramagnetic impurities, such as trivalent salts of iron or rare earth compounds, reduce the value of T_1 very significantly.

   To summarize, longitudinal relaxation is the process of building up the longitudinal component of the magnetization under the influence of the magnetic field $\mathbf{B_0}$. However, the field can generate magnetization only in its own direction. The stronger the $\mathbf{B_0}$ the larger the equilibrium magnetization M_∞. The approach to M_∞ is exponential and is described by a constant T_1, known as the longitudinal relaxation time.

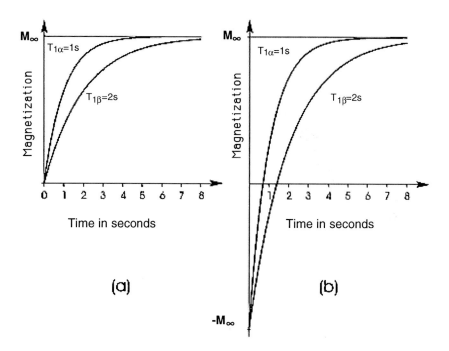

Figure 3.1. Longitudinal relaxation: the process by which magnetization attains the equilibrium value M_∞ starting from $M = 0$ (a). The time is counted from the moment of placing the object in the magnetic field. The two curves with different values of T_1 correspond to two different tissues, α and β. (b) Starting from $-M_\infty$, i.e. the situation when, after reaching M_∞, the magnetization was reversed using a π pulse (see Section 3.4). The time is counted from the moment the magnetization is rotated. In this case, the value of the magnetization passes through zero after a time $0.693T_1$ (strictly speaking $T_1 \ln 2$).

3.3 Larmor Precession

Magnetization created as a result of relaxation remains immobile in the direction of B_0, i.e. in the longitudinal direction. Compare this situation to a static swing. When displaced from the vertical position, the swing begins to oscillate periodically with a characteristic frequency. Similarly, magnetization displaced from its equilibrium position begins a periodic motion. The motion of the magnetization is somewhat different from that of a swing and more like a spinning top (Fig. 3.2a). In the course of this motion the magnetization moves along the surface of a cone, rotating in such a way that the angle between itself and B_0 is constant (Fig. 3.2b). This motion of the magnetization is known as the "Larmor precession", and the angle as the precession angle.

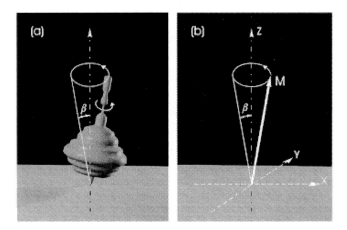

Figure 3.2. Precession. (a) A spinning top does not topple over, but rotates with its rotation axis precessing around the vertical direction. The axis of the top moves on the surface of a cone. The angle β between the axis of rotation and the axis of the cone is known as the precession angle. (b) During Larmor precession magnetization undergoes a similar motion around the longitudinal direction determined by B_0.

The similarity of the motions of the magnetization and the spinning top comes from the fact that both cases involve spinning masses subjected to a torsional force: exerted by the magnetic field B_0 on the magnetic moment of the nucleus and by the force of gravity on the top. The spinning mass responds with precessional motion. A fuller explanation of precession exceeds the scope of this book.

The angular velocity ω_0 of Larmor precession depends on the strength of the field $\mathbf{B}_0$ and on the gyromagnetic ratio γ, a quantity characteristic of each kind of nucleus. Angular velocity of Larmor precession in radians per second is

$$\omega_0 = \gamma \, \mathbf{B}_0 \qquad (3.1)$$

or, in full revolutions per second

$$\nu_0 = \frac{\gamma \, \mathbf{B}_0}{2\pi} . \qquad (3.1a)$$

For protons the ratio γ expressed in radians per second per tesla is 2.6752196×10^8. Eq. (3.1a) shows therefore that in a field of 1 tesla the magnetization of protons performs no fewer than 42577470 full revolutions per second. Gyromagnetic ratios of all nuclei with spin have been measured with enormous accuracy, and some of the values are given in Table 3.1.

Table 3.1. Frequencies of magnetic resonance and other properties of some isotopes.

Isotope	Natural abundance (%)	Resonance frequency in $B_0 = 1$ T field	
		ν_0 (Hz)	ω_0 (radians/second)
^{1}H	99.985	42.577×10^6	267.52×10^6
^{2}H	0.015	6.5360×10^6	41.067×10^6
^{13}C	1.10	10.7082×10^6	67.281×10^6
^{14}N	99.634	3.0779×10^6	19.339×10^6
^{15}N	0.366	4.3173×10^6	27.126×10^6
^{19}F	100.00	40.0777×10^6	251.81×10^6
^{23}Na	100.00	11.2690×10^6	70.805×10^6
^{31}P	100.00	17.2515×10^6	108.39×10^6

Depending on the kind of nucleus, Larmor precession can occur in the clockwise or the anticlockwise direction, but this is quite unimportant to MRI. Magnetization deflected from the longitudinal direction has a non-zero transverse component (Fig. 2.7). It is important to bear in mind that as a result of precession the transverse component rotates with the angular velocity ω_0 while the longitudinal component is static.

3.4 Nuclear Magnetic Resonance

How can one deflect the static vector of magnetization from the longitudinal direction and force it to precess? The answer is given in Fig. 3.3. The object "c" is placed inside a magnet and subjected to the action of the strong magnetic field $\mathbf{B_0}$. In the close vicinity of the object and perpendicular to $\mathbf{B_0}$ there is a small coil "b" known as the transmitter-receiver coil. The coil is connected to a source of electric current with frequency ω_e (the connection is not shown) generating a variable magnetic field. The oscillation of the field has the same frequency as the current:

$$2B_1 \cos \omega_e t \qquad (3.2)$$

where $2B_1$ is the amplitude of the oscillations.

The object is thus subjected to the action of *two* mutually perpendicular magnetic fields: the very strong constant field $\mathbf{B_0}$ and an oscillating field with amplitude $2B_1$ which is at least 10,000 times smaller. Under the action of the oscillating field the angle of precession changes continuously according to

$$\beta = \gamma B_1 \tau \qquad (3.3)$$

where τ is the time counted from the moment when the oscillating field is switched on. The change of the angle β which was initially zero is equivalent to the deflection of the magnetization from the longitudinal direction (Fig. 3.4).

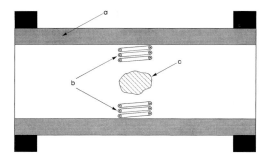

Figure 3.3. Schematic representation of an MRI spectrometer. (a) Coil generating a strong constant magnetic field B_o. (b) Transmitter-receiver coil which, when connected to a generator of alternating electric current of radiofrequency creates a weak variable magnetic field $2B_1 \cos \omega_e t$ in the direction perpendicular to B_o. (c) Object under study. When the magnetization of the object is made to precess by the alternating field impulse, the coil (b) is disconnected from the generator and connected to the receiver which observes the signal. The reconnection is done by a dedicated electronic device not shown in the Figure.

This method of deflecting the magnetization from the longitudinal direction is effective only when the oscillating field fulfils the following two conditions:

(a) Its direction is not parallel to B_o, and
(b) Its frequency is equal to the frequency of the precession, so that $\omega_e = \omega_o$.

In other words, the "resonance condition"

$$\omega_e = \gamma B_o \qquad (3.4)$$

must be satisfied. It follows that the magnetization can only be deflected by a field oscillating with a strictly determined frequency.

The action of the oscillating field is highly selective with respect to the kind of nucleus. The reason for this is that the values of the gyromagnetic ratios, and consequently of the resonance frequencies, for different nuclei are very different (see Table 3.1). It follows that when the generator is tuned to produce frequency ω_e which satisfies the resonance condition Eq. (3.4) for nuclei of one element, the magnetization of other atomic nuclei in the object is completely unaffected. In short, only magnetization of one kind of nuclei undergoes nuclear resonance and only this magnetization is made to precess.

Physical effects associated with one strictly determined frequency are conventionally known as resonance. This is why the deflection of the direction of the magnetization is properly known as Nuclear Magnetic Resonance (NMR). Medical literature omits the word "nuclear" as unfriendly, and uses the abbreviation MR instead. NMR was discovered in 1945 by two independent American research groups: the Harvard group led by E. M. Purcell and the Stanford group by F. Bloch. MRI was invented in 1973 simultaneously by the American scientist P. C. Lauterbur, who originally proposed the name "zeugmatography", and by the British physicist P. Mansfield.

The conditions of nuclear magnetic resonance stated as (a) and (b) above are rigorously justified by quantum mechanics. However, we can grasp the general idea of their meaning from the analogy with a swing. Note that:

(a) We cannot make the swing oscillate by pulling it downwards. The applied force must be perpendicular to the direction of gravity.

(b) The swing can be made to oscillate very vigorously even if pushed gently but repeatedly, provided that the successive strokes are applied at suitable equal time intervals, i.e. at the natural frequency of oscillation, then the effect of the individual strokes accumulates. This analogy explains why a very small variable field of resonance frequency is able to "take over" the magnetization from the much stronger field B_0.

To deflect the nuclear magnetization, the resonance condition Eq. (3.4) need not be satisfield absolutely precisely. There is a certain tolerance. When, as a result of inhomogeneity, the field in one region of the object is B_0 and in another region $B_0 + \delta$, the variable magnetic field of amplitude $2B_1$ and frequency $\omega_e = \gamma B_0$ may deflect the magnetization by the same angle in both regions at once, as long as δ is much smaller than $2B_1$. If one considers that the amplitude $2B_1$ is ca. 10,000 times smaller than B_0, this tolerance is quite low. However, as we shall see in Section 4.1, it is crucial to MRI. A fuller discussion of the reasons for this effect exceeds the scope of this book.

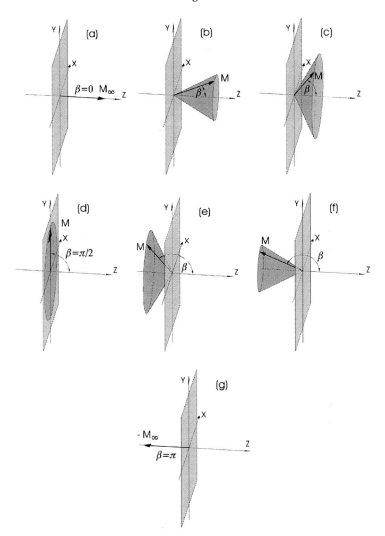

Figure 3.4. Continuous change of the precession angle under the influence of the oscillating magnetic field of resonance frequency $\omega_e = \gamma\, B_o$ and amplitude $2B_1$. The process is continuous according to $\beta = \gamma\, B_1\, \tau$, but the Figure shows only several distinct stages. (a) Initial stage with $\beta = 0$; (b)–(c) Increase of the angle β; (d) $\beta = \pi/2$ when the cone of precession coincides with the plane perpendicular to B_o; (e)–(f) Further increase of the angle β; (g) $\beta = \pi$ when the magnetization is inverted to point in the opposite direction to B_o. If the process continues, the magnetization will return to the position (a) passing sequentially through stages (f), (e) etc. The process can be interrupted at any time by switching off the alternating field, whereupon the magnetization will precess preserving the angle β which it has reached. The Z axis coincides with the direction of the constant magnetic field B_o.

In practice, in MRI and in other applications of nuclear magnetic resonance the object under examination is subjected to the action of the high-frequency magnetic field only for a very short period, of the order of 1/1000 of a second. It receives a "radiofrequency pulse". The pulse is administered by a computer-driven device which electronically switches the alternating current on and off. During the pulse the precession angle reaches a certain value which remains constant after the pulse ceases. This angle can be calculated from Eq. (3.3) if τ is treated as the duration of the pulse.

A pulse which forces the magnetization to precess with the precession angle $\beta = \pi/2$ is known as a $\pi/2$ pulse. Such a pulse moves the magnetization from the position shown in Fig. 3.4a to the position in Fig. 3.4d. In other words, a $\pi/2$ pulse rotates the magnetization, so far aligned with $\mathbf{B}_0$, by the angle $\pi/2$ thus placing it in the transverse plane, so that further precession takes place in that plane.

A pulse which rotates the magnetization by the angle π, i.e. moves it from position (a) to position (g) in Fig. 3.4 is known as a π pulse. The π pulse merely reverses the sense of the magnetization vector, leaving it aligned with the –Z axis. $\pi/2$ and π pulses are often used in MRI.

The present discussion of the behaviour of the magnetization disregards the process of relaxation, focusing attention on what happens to the magnetization during and immediately after the pulse, i.e. over less than 0.001 of a second. This is entirely justified because relaxation in the various tissues of the human body is relatively slow. For relaxation effects to be perceptible we would have to wait much longer, for at least 0.1 of a second.

3.5 Free Induction Decay

We already know that every magnetic moment generates lines of magnetic field. This also applies to the total magnetic moment of an assembly of many atomic nuclei. Following a $\pi/2$ pulse the lines of field of the precessing magnetization criss-cross the coils of the transmitter-receiver coil thus generating an oscillating voltage (Fig. 3.5) by Faraday's electromagnetic induction. The induced voltage is known as the "Free Induction Decay" (abbreviated as FID), and is measured by disconnecting the coil from the frequency generator immediately after the pulse and connecting it to a receiver. The FID is generated also by pulses other than the $\pi/2$ pulse, but with a lower amplitude.

The FID decays with time (Fig. 3.5) because of the decrease of the transverse magnetization. The tip of the vector of transverse magnetization moves not on the circumference of a circle, but on a spiral running towards the centre of the circle. This "transverse relaxation" has a different time constant from the time constant T_1 of longitudinal relaxation, known as the transverse relaxation time T_2. Unlike longitudinal relaxation which drives the longitudinal component towards M_∞, the limiting value of the transverse component is zero.

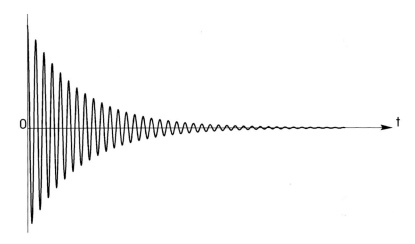

Figure 3.5. Free induction decay (FID) of frequency $\omega_0 = \gamma \, B_0$ following the application of a pulse. The amplitude of the FID is maximum when a $\pi/2$ pulse is applied.

We see therefore that the motions of the longitudinal and transverse components are independent of one another and follow different laws. This is why it is more useful to consider the vector of magnetization in terms of its longitudinal and transverse components rather than as a single entity. While the longitudinal component M_z approaches M_∞ on the T_1 timescale, the transverse component $M_\perp$ precesses at the frequency ω_0 and decreases towards zero with another time constant, T_2. Independent changes of the components determine the behaviour of the magnetization as a whole and finally reach equilibrium at which $M_z = M_\infty$ and $M_\perp = 0$.

The decay of the transverse component is caused by two factors: magnetic interactions between nuclei and the inhomogeneity of the field B_0. The first of these is of a quantum nature and will not be discussed here. The second reason can be understood by reference to magnetization expressed as a sum of partial magnetizations (isochromats) coming from different regions of the object and subjected to different strengths of the field B_0. These precess with slightly different frequencies. Although initially, just after the pulse, the isochromats are parallel to one another (i.e. precess together with the same phase), after a time they "fan out" as shown in Fig. 3.6. This process shortens their vector sum and causes the induced signal to decay.

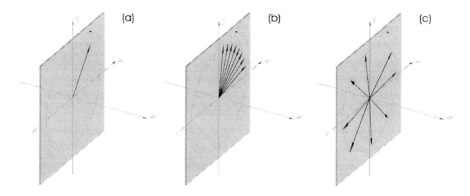

Figure 3.6. The "fanning out" of the magnetization. (a) Immediately after a $\pi/2$ pulse all the components of the magnetization (isochromats) coming from all segments of the object under study precess with the same phase in the transverse plane. A strong signal is then induced in the transmitted-receiver coil. (b) As time passes, as a result of the inhomogeneity of field B_0 some isochromats precess faster and some slower. The resultant magnetization (vector sum) decreases. (c) After some time the isochromats are evenly distributed in all directions on the transverse plane. The resultant magnetization is zero and the signal disappears. The process which causes the damping of the signal is governed by the time constant T_2^*.

When the field B_0 is highly homogeneous, the quantum mechanism (internuclear interaction) dominates and the transverse relaxation time is denoted by T_2. Conversely, when the rate of relaxation is mainly determined by the inhomogeneity of the field, we stress this by using the symbol T_2^*. Transverse magnetization in the same object placed in a homogeneous field decays with the time constant T_2, and placed in an inhomogeneous field with the time constant T_2^*. Since in the latter case field inhomogeneity is an additional relaxation mechanism, the time T_2^* may be considerably shorter than T_2. Normally T_2 is shorter than T_1 even in homogeneous fields. In human tissues both these quantities have values between 100 and 2500 ms.

Appropriate manipulation of pulses and field gradients can reverse the effects of relaxation caused by field inhomogeneity (see Section 3.6). On the other hand, the decay of the magnetization caused by internuclear interactions is irreversible. Magnetization cannot be quickly brought back to its original value if the decay occurred in this way. The only solution is to wait for equilibrium to be established and send the magnetization into the transverse plane again. We thus refer to irreversible transverse relaxation (governed by the time T_2) and (at least partially) reversible relaxation (governed by T_2^*).

3.6 Spin Echo

Consider a situation in which the main reason for the decay of the FID is the inhomogeneity of the field $\mathbf{B_0}$. The slower components of the "fan" of partial magnetizations drag behind the faster components (Figs. 3.6b and 3.7b). A π pulse will act on the transverse magnetizations in the same way as on the longitudinal component: each individual partial magnetization will rotate by 180°. The result is the reversal of the order of partial magnetizations in the fan: those which precessed faster are now behind the slower ones (Fig. 3.7c) and begin to "catch up" with them. After a certain time the fan is again folded into a single vector. The signal generated in the receiver coil as a result of this process is known as the "spin echo" (Fig. 3.7a).

The π pulse does not affect the rate of the precession, which depends only on the magnitude of the field $\mathbf{B_0}$ in which a given partial magnetization precesses. This is why the rate of "folding" of the fan is exactly the same as the rate at which it "unfolds" during the time τ between the $\pi/2$ pulse and the π pulse. The maximum of the echo is thus at 2τ counting from the $\pi/2$ pulse. It is usual to denote the appearance of the echo maximum by the symbol TE ("echo time"), so that TE = 2τ.

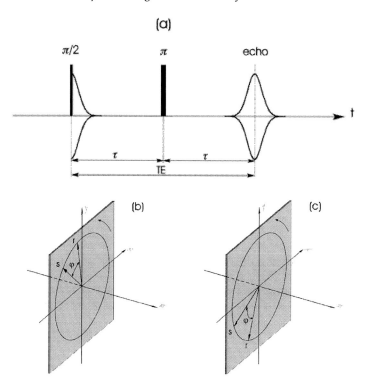

Figure 3.7. Spin echo. (a) The course of the experiment: After equilibrium has been reached, a $\pi/2$ pulse is applied to the object. The FID (of which only the envelope is drawn) decreases very rapidly because of the inhomogeneity of the magnetic field. After time τ, when the signal has disappeared, a π pulse is applied. After another τ interval the object by itself induces a signal known as the spin echo. (b) Situation just before the π pulse is applied (only two isochromats are shown for clarity). The angle φ between the isochromats arose during time τ as a result of field inhomogeneity. (c) Situation just after the application of the π pulse. The angle φ is the same, but the order of the isochromats has changed: the fast isochromat (f) is now behind the slow isochromat (s) and will "catch up" with it after exactly the same time τ which was needed to create the angle φ. The fast, slow and other isochromats come together after the time TE = 2τ counting from the $\pi/2$ pulse to give the echo signal.

The cause of the growth and the decay of the spin echo is the same: the inhomogeneity of the field $\mathbf{B}_0$. This is why the echo takes the form of two FIDs combined back-to-back. Were it not for the irreversible relaxation caused by internuclear interactions (see Section 3.5), the maximum amplitude of the echo would in principle be equal to the original amplitude of the FID. The time τ (= 1/2TE) may be set by the operator a t will.   If TE is much shorter than T_2, the damping of the echo is insignificant, otherwise the height of the echo is determined by irreversible damping. This effect makes spin echo useful for MRI (see Section 4.3).

The π pulse can generate the spin echo because the orientation of partial magnetizations immediately after the $\pi/2$ pulse is parallel. This is also the case at the top of the echo. It follows that when another π pulse is applied after the echo, a second echo will appear. This effect is used in localized spectroscopy (see Section 4.3).

In another method of obtaining the spin echo, the π pulse is not applied. It can be used when the inhomogeneity of the magnetic field is caused only by the gradient coils. Instead of applying the π pulse, the direction of the field gradient is suddenly reversed by reversing the direction of the current in the gradient coils. The partial magnetizations which were exposed to a stronger field before the direction of the gradient was reversed, find themselves in a weaker field, and vice versa. Thus after TE = 2τ all partial magnetizations come together with the same phase and induce a signal in the receiver coil known as the gradient echo.

CHAPTER 4

IMAGING

4.1 Experimental Procedure

MRI works on the principle of imaging thin slices of objects. The individual body organs are distinguishable in the image because different tissues have different abilities to induce magnetic resonance signals. We shall discuss the principles of the experimental procedure in some detail.

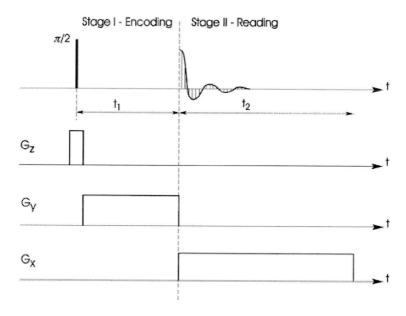

Figure 4.1. The course of a "single experiment" which, repeated many times with different values of time t_1, provides the data necessary for the creation of an MRI image. The sequence of events in the experiment is as follows. A $\pi/2$ pulse applied in the presence of a G_z gradient stimulates the chosen slice of the object. A G_y gradient is then applied, which after time t_1 (encoding time – Stage I) is replaced by a G_x gradient. The signal is sampled in the presence of the G_x gradient (reading time – Stage II).

41

A slice of the object uder study is selected by a $\pi/2$ pulse acting in tandem with the G_z gradient. The profile of the strength of the field $\mathbf{B_o}$ with the gradient is drawn in the lower part of Fig. 1.2. The upper part of the Figure shows the slice selected by a pulse of frequency ω_e. The magnitude of the field satisfies the resonance condition only in a slice perpendicular to the Z axis for which

$$\omega_e = \gamma \, \mathbf{B}_e$$

where ω_e is the frequency of the pulse and γ the gyromagnetic ratio of the nuclei which give rise to the image. In the present state of MRI these are almost always protons. The pulse has no effect on the magnetization outside the selected slice.

Immediately following the $\pi/2$ pulse, the G_z gradient gives way to the G_y gradient for time t_1. This is in turn replaced by the G_x gradient which persists until the end of the FID. The duration t_1 of the G_y gradient, during which no actual measurement is performed, is the "encoding time". The duration t_2 of the G_x gradient, during which the FID is sampled, is the "read time", and the G_x gradient itself is known as the "read gradient". The whole sequence, known as a "single experiment", is schematically shown in Fig. 4.1.

The data are gathered by repeating the single experiment many times, each time with a different value of t_1. If a single experiment samples the FID m times, then after n experiments there are $n \times m$ results which are a table of values of the function $f(t_1, t_2)$. There are two time variables, because each measurement corresponds to the values of t_1 *and* t_2 with which it was performed. In successive experiments the duration t_1 of the G_y gradient is increased stepwise, for example from 0.05 ms to 12.8 ms in 0.05 ms steps (1 ms = 1/1000 of a second). Sampling over time t_2 is done in identical steps. The values of n and m (which may be equal or different) determine the resolution of the image. Typical values are 128 $(= 2^7)$ or 256 $(= 2^8)$. Since the precise values are unimportant to the principle of the experiment, we shall assume that $n = m$. For example, with $n = m = 256$ the number of results is $256 \times 256 = 2^{16} = 65536$, so that a powerful computer workstation is needed to register and transform the results from which the brightness of the individual elements of the image is calculated. The treatment of data is described Section 4.2.

After the end of a single experiment no magnetization remains in the slice: the longitudinal component has been cancelled by the $\pi/2$ pulse, and the transverse component has decayed with the FID. It follows that we need to wait for a certain time to allow longitudinal magnetization to recover sufficiently via longitudinal relaxation before embarking on another experiment. The time between the $\pi/2$ pulse which initiates a single experiment and the $\pi/2$ pulse which initiates the next is the "repetition time" TR.

4.2 Transformation of the Results

In Section 4.1 we described a series of measurements with different values of t_1 and t_2 which produces a total of n^2 results. These will be refered to collectively as $f(t_1, t_2)$ and treated as a table of values of a function of two variables. In order to build an image of the slice we need to calculate the intensities of the signals induced by its individual elements.

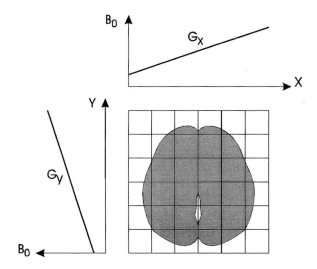

Figure 4.2. Division of the chosen slice into columns and rows. The plot on the left shows the distribution of of the strength of B_0 along the Y axis (gradient G_y) during encoding, and the plot at the top shows the strength of B_0 along the X axis (gradient G_x) during sampling. As a result of these successive gradients the slice is divided first into rows and then into columns. In practice a slice is divided into a much larger number of rows and columns.

Imagine that the slice is divided into n columns and n rows, a total of n^2 elements (see Fig. 4.2). The magnetization of nuclei in an individual element is known as "partial magnetization". At the second stage of a single experiment, i.e. while the G_x gradient is applied, the magnetic field increases along the X axis, so that each column experiences a slightly different field $\mathbf{B_o}$. This discriminates between the columns on the basis of the induced frequency which is directly proportional to the strength of the field ($\omega = \gamma \mathbf{B}$). Thus there is a strict relationship between the frequency and the spatial location of each column. For example, we can refer to a column as "column ω_2" if the frequency of the signal induced by this column during Stage II is ω_2. Similarly, during Stage I the G_y gradient discriminates between the individual rows, and we can refer to a row as "row ω_1" if the frequency of the signal induced by this row is ω_1. Thus the G_y and G_x gradients unmistakably identify each element of the slice in terms of two frequencies: precession frequency ω_1 during Stage I and precession frequency ω_2 during Stage II.

Information about frequency ω_1 can be obtained even though there was no sampling during Stage I. This is because the precession of elementary magnetizations during Stage I also affects the signal measured during Stage II. We can say that Stage I prepares Stage II, which begins when the G_y gradient is replaced by the G_x gradient. The signal depends on the phase of the precessional motion of partial magnetizations at the moment when the gradient direction was changed, i.e. at $t_2 = 0$. The partial magnetizations continue to precesss during Stage II, starting with these phases, but at a different frequency. The phase at $t_2 = 0$ depends on ω_1 and t_1: the frequency of precession and the length of Stage I. Therefore information about precession during Stage I is "encoded" in the form of the various phases and transferred to Stage II. Accordingly, Stage I is known as the time of "phase encoding".

In order to pick out the signals from the individual elements and determine their amplitudes we subject the function $f(t_1, t_2)$ to the mathematical treatment known as two-dimensional Fourier transformation, similar to the ordinary (one-dimensional) Fourier transformation described in Chapter 2. The difference is that two-dimensional transformation is applied to functions of two variables. They are not decomposed into a sum of individual cosines but into a sum of products of two cosines with a common amplitude $F(\omega_1, \omega_2)$

$$F(\omega_1, \omega_2) \cos \omega_1 t_1 \cos \omega_2 t_2 .$$

These functions describe the motion of the magnetization in the individual elements of the slice: with frequency ω_1 during Stage I and frequency ω_2 during Stage II. The amplitude $F(\omega_1, \omega_2)$ thus describes the intensities of signals induced by the individual elements. The computer displays these elements on the screen with brightness proportional to $F(\omega_1, \omega_2)$, thus producing the image of the slice.

The two-dimensional Fourier transformation can be understood by reference to the one-dimensional version (see Section 2.3). Consider a particular single experiment. The results of sampling $f(\bar{t}_1, t_2)$ are a function of time t_2, while for this experiment the value of $\bar{t}_1$ is fixed, which is stressed with the horizontal bar above. The function $f(\bar{t}_1, t_2)$ is thus a function of just one variable t_2 and can be Fourier transformed in one dimension using the familiar procedure. In this way we decompose the measured signal into columns, and arrive at the function $F(\bar{t}_1, \omega_2)$ which describes the amplitudes of signals coming from the individual columns. By repeating this calculation for each single experiment we obtain a function of two variables $F(t_1, \omega_2)$ where t_1 (without a horizontal bar) goes through the values used in the single experiments, and ω_2 through the frequencies corresponding to the individual columns.

Consider now a single column, say column $\bar{\omega}_2$. The function $F(t_1, \bar{\omega}_2)$ gives us the amplitudes of signals for this column in the single experiments described by t_1. It is a function of only one variable t_1 and can be Fourier transformed in one dimension. The transformation decomposes the signal from this column into frequencies induced by its elements. The result is the function $F(\omega_1, \bar{\omega}_2)$. By repeating the same transformations for each individual column we arrive at the function $F(\omega_1, \omega_2)$ corresponding to the brightness of the individual elements of the image.

Two-dimensional Fourier transformation consists therefore of sequential application of two one-dimensional transformations: first with respect to one variable and then with respect to the other. Although the first transformation in the above example was with respect to the variable t_2 and the second with respect to t_1, the order is unimportant for the final result.

Note that if the FID was also sampled during Stage I and the signals from both stages separately Fourier transformed in one dimension, only information about whole columns and whole rows would be obtained. Such information does not reveal the status of the individual elements.

The above is only one of many methods of two-dimensional nuclear magnetic resonance spectroscopy. The idea of the two-dimensional experiment was first suggested in 1971 by J. Jeener with a view to chemical applications. Soon after, A. Kumar, D. Welti and R. R. Ernst pointed out that two-dimensional Fourier transformation may be useful in MRI. Lauterbur, the inventor of magnetic resonance imaging, used a method known as "projection reconstruction". Although this is still in use, the most frequently used method nowadays is a variant of the Kumar, Welti and Ernst experiment, in which the echo signal is sampled (see Section 4.3). Yet another method, "Echo Planar Imaging", introduced by Mansfield, is particularly fast because single experiments need not be repeated. Sampling is done in only one specially designed experiment.

4.3 Contrast Adjustment

The MRI image is a map of signal intensity. As we know, signal intensity depends on several factors, such as the number of protons per unit volume of tissue (the "proton density"), and the relaxation times T_1 and T_2. We will now show how the contribution of one of these factors can be emphasised at the expense of other contributions, so as to obtain the image "weighted" towards this factor. The term implies that the influence of the remaining factors is not entirely eliminated.

A "T_1-weighted" image is obtained as follows. We know that after the completion of each single experiment no magnetization is left in the slice. This means that we have to wait for a certain time (known as the "waiting time") to allow longitudinal relaxation to restore the magnetization, at least partially, to its equilibrium value. Otherwise the $\pi/2$ pulse in the next single experiment will have no magnetization to rotate and no signal will appear. The waiting time must be the same for the entire series of single experiments, otherwise the relative intensities from the different elements of the image would be incorrect. The waiting time depends on the distance between the $\pi/2$ pulses belonging to successive single experiments, i.e. on the "repetition time" TR. This is controlled by the electronic circuits and can be set to any value.

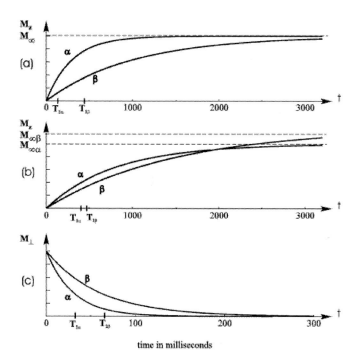

Figure 4.3. Comparison of the course of relaxation in tissues α and β. (a) Longitudinal relaxation when $T_{1\alpha} < T_{1\beta}$ and the proton densities are equal. The largest difference occurs when the delay time is close to $T_{1\alpha}$ and $T_{1\beta}$. (b) Longitudinal relaxation when $T_{1\alpha} < T_{1\beta}$ and the proton density of tissue β is larger than that of tissue α. A delay time close to $T_{1\alpha}$ and $T_{1\beta}$ will give a stronger signal for tissue α, and a very long delay time a stronger signal for tissue β. (c) Transverse relaxation for $T_{2\alpha} < T_{2\beta}$ and equal proton density in both tissues.

In order to see how the value of TR affects the contrast between two tissues we examine the recovery curves of longitudinal magnetization M_z. Fig. 4.3 shows these curves for various relaxation times as well as the proton density of two tissues: tissue α and tissue β. Fig. 4.3a applies to the case when the proton density in both tissues is the same but the relaxation times differ, so that $T_{1\alpha} < T_{1\beta}$. Equal proton densities mean that the magnetizations of both tissues approach the same limiting value M_∞. This process of longitudinal relaxation (see Section 3.2) proceeds faster in tissue α which has a shorter relaxation time. The different relaxation times make the curves grow further apart in the interval between $T_{1\alpha}$ and $T_{1\beta}$.

The magnitude of magnetization with which each tissue enters the next single experiment depends on the moment at which the $\pi/2$ pulse of this experiment appears. If at this moment the relaxation curves are far apart, the strength of signals from different tissues will be different, thus increasing the contrast of the image. If the curves are close together, the contrast is low. It follows that waiting times close to $T_{1\alpha}$ and $T_{1\beta}$ result in the greatest contrast.

Fig. 4.3b illustrates the case of two tissues with different T_1 relaxation times and different proton densities. The tissue with longer T_1 relaxation time is marked with β. When the proton density in this tissue is lower, the curves do not cross. However, a longer waiting time gives a "proton density-weighted" image and a shorter waiting time a T_1-weighted image.

There is one more method, known as "Inversion Recovery" (IR), which makes very good use of the different T_1 in different tissues. Inversion Recovery uses very long repetition times which allow the magnetization to reach the equilibrium value M_∞ after each single experiment. A π pulse is then applied before the $\pi/2$ pulse normally initiating the next single experiment. The π pulse rotates the magnetization by 180° (see Section 3.4), which then begins to relax starting from the value $-M_\infty$ and tends towards M_∞ as shown in Fig. 3.1b. In this procedure the differences in T_1 of the various tissues are much more pronounced than when relaxation begins from zero, which increases the contrast of the image. In addition, Inversion Recovery allows the signal from any chosen tissue to be extinguished. Let $T_{1\alpha}$ stand for the relaxation time of such a tissue. If the time delay between π and $\pi/2$ pulses (often denoted by TIR) is chosen so that TIR $= 0.693\,T_{1\alpha}$, the $\pi/2$ pulse will have nothing to rotate in this tissue, because its magnetization is zero exactly at the moment this pulse is applied. In other words, in the chosen tissue the $\pi/2$ pulse will not generate the transverse magnetization necessary for the MRI signal to appear. The application of Inversion Recovery is illustrated in Fig. 5.13, where the signal from the cerebrospinal fluid is extinguished in the image of a transverse section of the brain.

The transverse relaxation times T_2 of tissues may differ quite substantially (Fig. 4.3c). In order to use this for achieving contrast we resort to the spin echo, the signal which depends on T_2. Since the method which gives T_1-weighted images does not generate a spin echo, we use the single experiment shown in Fig. 4.4. The G_x gradient is applied for the

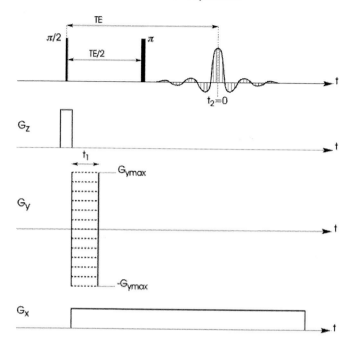

Figure 4.4. Single experiment with spin echo, used for creating T_2-weighted images. For details see Section 4.3.

entire duration of the experiment, even when the G_y gradient is applied. The encoding time t_1 is constant, but the G_y gradient is varied in small increments between one experiment and another. In fact, since the phase of the various magnetizations at the instant the G_y gradient ceases depends on the product $t_1 \times G_y$, it does not matter in principle whether it is t_1 or G_y which is changed. In consecutive single experiments the G_y gradient varies stepwise between fixed limits $-G_{ymax}$ and $+G_{ymax}$. The π pulse given at an arbitrarily chosen time TE/2 following the G_y gradient induces the echo with a maximum at time TE. The measured echo signal is a function of two variables: time t_2 and the value of the gradient G_y. Since, unlike in the case of the FID, it is impossible to determine with any precision when the echo begins, the time t_2 is counted from the moment TE when the echo is at a maximum. The image is obtained by Fourier transforming the echo signal in two dimensions, G_y and t_2. The use of the echo instead of the FID does not change the principle of how the image is acquired, because the information content of the two kinds of signals is the same: the echo is composed of two back-to-back FID signals (see Section 3.6). The use of constant t_1 enables the same value of TE to be used in all single experiments. The intensity of the echo is then equally affected by the transverse (T_2) relaxation.

Fig. 4.3c shows that the largest difference between the signals from two tissues with transverse relaxation times $T_{2\alpha}$ and $T_{2\beta}$ is obtained when TE is close to $T_{2\alpha}$ and $T_{2\beta}$. Short TE reduces the influence of transverse relaxation, while it would be pointless to use long TE because it gives low intensity signals.

Spin echo imaging makes it possible to control the contrast by adjusting either the TE or the waiting time. T_2- and T_1-weighted images may therefore be obtained, which opens wide possibilities for different diagnostic problems. The fact that optimum contrast can be achieved in different ways, without administering contrast-enhancing chemicals to the patient is an important advantage of MRI.

We have seen that the basic MRI method can be modified in different ways. The aim of the modifications is to bring out the details of the image which are important for the correct diagnosis. The following sections describe two further modifications.

The contrast depends not only on factors which are under the operator's control, but to a certain extent also onthe strength of the magnetic field B_o, which is constant for a given piece of equipment. It turns out that the difference between the relaxation times is normally higher in low fields (say 0.3 T) than in high fields (such as 1.5 T). On the other hand, the important advantage of strong fields is the increased signal-to-noise ratio, which makes the measurements faster, and therefore counts in the economics of the imager in the longer term. Since the cost of the equipment increases steeply with the strength of the magnetic field, the compromise field is around 1T, provided we do not plan to use localized spectroscopy (Section 4.6) which requires 1.5 or even 2 T fields. Incidentally, 2 T is the highest field permitted for hospital use in the United States. All the same, a number of imagers with 3 and 4 T fields are used for research on "functional analysis" which studies the function of the various parts of the brain. Even stronger fields are used in microimagers for examining small objects, not necessarily of medical interest. Fig. 5.18 shows the image of the abdomen of a drone bee taken in a 6.4 T field.

4.4 Contrast Agents

Sometimes lesions of interest to the clinician do not show a significant difference of T_1 and T_2 relaxation times from normal tissues and are not well discriminated. In such cases it can be helpful to administer a contrast agent, a substance which enhances the relaxation rate differentially. One such agent is an aqueous solution of the gadolinium chelate Gd DTPA (DTPA = diethylenetriamine pentaacetic acid). Gadolinium, a rare earth element, has a strong electronic magnetic moment coming from its unpaired $4f$ electrons. Unfortunately, the salts of gadolinium are poisonous. However, the chelate engages the valence electrons of the Ga ion and renders the molecule unreactive and non-toxic. In this form gadolinium is tolerated by the body. After ca. 12 hours of intravenous administration the complex accumulates in the kidneys and is removed in the urine. By interacting magnetically with the protons, the contrast agent shortens the relaxation times of protons in its vicinity. If the agent goes preferentially to the lesion, it causes it to show up with improved contrast.

Contrast agents penetrate the tissues with the blood and shorten T_1 and T_2 in various ways. This effect is used to generate T_2- or T_1-weighted images with better contrast and greater diagnostic value. Contrast agents are sometimes very helpful, for example for imaging the disorders of the blood-brain barrier. The contrast agent penetrates the lesion membrane, but the large chelate group is unable to penetrate the blood-brain barrier. Contrast agents thus make it possible to image the inflamed layer which normally surrounds a morbid growth. In this way the extent of a tumour may be precisely determined.

4.5 MRI Angiography

MRI angiography images only the cardiovascular system and disregards other organs of the body. The technique uses the flow of blood to obtain very strong contrast between blood and the static tissues. The information it provides is of considerable value to medical diagnostics.

Several variants of MRI angiography are in use. The principle of the simplest of them is to use very short waiting time in comparison with the T_1 of the tissues. As we know from Section 4.3, immobile tissues do not give a signal in this case because the magnetization has no time to recover

between the single experiments.   However, with flowing blood the
situation is different.   Fig. 4.5a shows the situation immediately after a
$\pi/2$ pulse in a slice traversing a blood vessel.   The pulse sends the
magnetization into the transverse plane; the longitudinal component
ceases to exist.   The zero magnetization of the slice is marked by hatching.

(a)

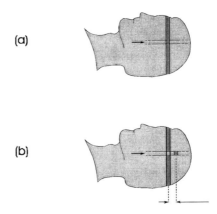

(b)

Figure 4.5. Principle of flow angiography (TOF).   The Figure shows a slice of the body and a
blood vessel passing through it.   Shaded area represents material with no longitudinal
magnetization. (a) Situation immediately after the $\pi/2$ pulse. (b) Situation at the end of the
delay period, i.e. just before the application of the next $\pi/2$ pulse.

Fig. 4.5b shows the same slice just before the $\pi/2$ pulse of the next
single experiment.   Since the waiting time is short, all the elements of the
slice are still unmagnetized with the exception of the region of flowing
blood.   This is because the blood which had no magnetization has already
left the slice and was replaced by a new portion of blood from outside the
slice.   Only this newly arrived blood carries longitudinal magnetization
which can give rise to the signal in the second single experiment.   The same
situation is present between successive single experiments.   As a result a
bright spot appears on the image at the location of the blood vessel and all
other elements of the image are dark.   This imaging method is known as
"time of flight" (TOF) angiography.

In order to obtain the image of blood vessels in a certain region of the body, for example the brain, we use this principle to take images of many closely spaced slices. The computer can create a spatial map of the blood vessels from the information on where blood vessels cross the successive layers. Time of flight angiography can also be used to measure the rate of blood flow. The problem reduces to finding the distance $\Delta\ell$ covered by non-magnetized blood during the waiting time Δt. The velocity of blood is then

$$v = \frac{\Delta\ell}{\Delta t} \, .$$

The distance $\Delta\ell$ can be determined by performing alternate single experiments for two slices. If the distance between the slices is $\Delta\ell$, blood in one of them will give no signal. In addition, the direction of blood flow can be determined.

Another method of visualizing blood vessels uses the spin echo. Nuclear magnetic moments in flowing blood travel in the centre of the blood vessel at a different velocity than close to its walls. As a result, in the presence of the field gradient the moving nuclear magnetic moments spend different amounts of time in regions with different values of the field B_0. This creates a certain disorder in the phase of precession, which in turn weakens the echo. This effect can be compensated for by appropriate gradient pulses without affecting the magnitude of signals from static tissues. If we take two images of the same slice, one with and one without compensation, and subtract one from the other, the intensity from the static tissues will cancel out but the blood will give a non-zero difference. The image will show only the blood vessels.

MRI angiography is distinct from methods which image blood vessels using X-rays or ultrasound. Its advantages are the very clear images and the fact that the technique does not require the use of contrast agents.

4.6 Localized Spectroscopy

Localized spectroscopy is a combination of MRI with high-resolution nuclear magnetic resonance spectroscopy (NMR), a technique which has been enormously successful in various areas of chemistry.

Soon after the discovery of magnetic resonance it was found that the precise resonance frequency of nuclei of the same isotope of the same element immersed in the same magnetic field B_0 depends to a very small degree on the kind of molecule in which the nucleus is found. Even nuclei of the same element in the same molecule may resonate at slightly different frequencies. This dependence of the resonance frequency of a nucleus on its chemical environment, and the frequency difference itself, are known as the "chemical shift". The set of resonances from a given substance is known as the spectrum.

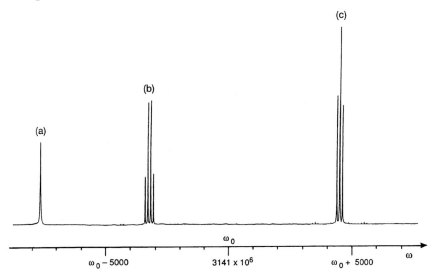

Figure 4.6. Nuclear magnetic resonance spectrum of protons in ethanol, CH_3–CH_2–OH in a 11.7433 T magnetic field. As a result of the chemical shift, the resonances in the individual groups correspond to different frequencies in the (a) OH group, (b) CH_2 group and (c) CH_3 group. The splitting of lines within groups is caused by the so-called electron-mediated spin-spin interaction.

The individual resonances appear in the spectrum as "lines". Consider, for example, the proton spectrum of ethyl alcohol, CH_3-CH_2-OH, a relatively simple organic compound (Fig. 4.6). A distinct group of spectral lines corresponds to each functional group in the molecule. The distance between the families of lines on the frequency scale is the chemical shift and the splitting within the individual groups is caused by yet another effect, known as spin-spin coupling. Both depend on the three-dimensional structure of the molecule. The spectrum distinguishes a given compound from other molecules, thus becoming a tool of qualitative analysis, and provides information about its molecular structure. From the intensity of the various spectral lines we can determine the ratio of intensities of the individual components of a mixture, which is an important tool of quantitative analysis. Interpretation of nuclear magnetic resonance spectra is an extensive field straddling the boundary of physics and chemistry.

A high-resolution spectrum is obtained by measuring the FID in a homogeneous magnetic field. The FID is Fourier transformed and the spectrum is simply the plot of the Fourier transform $F(\omega)$ of the signal. Two conditions must be satisfied for a high-resolution spectrum (a spectrum in which the individual resonances are clearly resolved) to be obtained. First, the magnetic field must be very homogeneous, otherwise the spectral lines will broaden and overlap. Second, the molecules under study must be in rapid thermal motion, as is the case in liquids and solutions. This condition is generally satisfied in tissues.

The cause of the chemical shift is the electronic currents induced in the electron shells of molecules by the magnetic field. These currents generate weak magnetic fields, which differ in different regions of the molecule. Those influence the value of the field experienced by the individual nuclei, and thus the frequency of the Larmor precession. The magnitude of the chemical shift is directly proportional to the strength of the field B_0, so that very high resolution spectra require strong magnetic fields.

Localized spectroscopy measures high-resolution spectra from a given region of the MRI image. This allows the operator to monitor the kind and concentration of metabolites in the tissue of interest.

In the simplest version of localized spectroscopy a selected volume element of the tissue is made to produce the second echo which is then Fourier transformed. As we know from Section 3.6, the second echo appears following three pulses: $\pi/2$, π and π. The gradients are manipulated in such a way that only the chosen volume resonates. If the G_z gradient is present for the duration of the $\pi/2$ pulse, the pulse will select a slice perpendicular to the Z axis (see Section 4.1). The π pulse together with the G_y gradient will select a slice perpendicular to the Y axis: the magnetization can be rotated by 180° only in this slice. The final π pulse together with the G_x pulse affects only a slice perpendicular to the X axis.

Only the volume belonging to all three slices at once will experience all three pulses and only this volume will produce the second echo. The signal appears after the gradients have been switched off, i.e. when the field is again homogeneous. The signal thus contains only those frequencies which correspond to different chemical shifts. The spectrum is obtained by subjecting the signal to one-dimensional Fourier transformation. In practice the region of which the spectrum is measured is selected by the operator guided by the image on the screen. The computer calculates the pulse frequencies required, thereby determining the position of the slices. Spectra of nuclei other than protons can also be measured.

Localized spectroscopy, also known as spatially selective spectroscopy, is an *in vivo* technique and studies undisturbed living cells.

CHAPTER 5

PRACTICAL ASPECTS

5.1 Specimen Images

This section gives a number of illustrative examples of the capabilities and potential of MRI, and of its practical use in medical diagnosis. The following abbreviations are used in the Figure captions :

MR	(Nuclear) magnetic resonance.
SE	Spin echo, and an image obtained with spin echo.
TR	Repetition time of "single experiments".
TE	The time after which spin echo appears, counting from the $\pi/2$ pulse.
TIR	Time delay between π and $\pi/2$ pulses in the Inversion Recovery method.
MRA	Magnetic resonance angiography.
MRA TOF	Time-of-flight magnetic resonance angiography.

The images in Figs. 5.1–5.11 were taken in a 0.5 T magnetic field with a Resonex Rx 5000HP imager, and contain 256 rows and 192 columns.

These images demonstrate the usefulness of MRI for the study of various anatomical structures, often enabling conclusions to be drawn about pathology. For example, Fig. 5.7 uses T_2-weighted images of the brain to reveal foci of variable size in the white matter of the brain. MRI is particularly useful when it allows the clinician access to anatomical structures which earlier required invasive radiological examination, such as administration of an iodide contrast agent followed by CT scanning. Fig. 5.14 shows the course of the acoustic nerve within the petrous temporal bone. Time-of-flight angiography is also non-invasive, and does not require catheterizing blood vessels or administration of contrast agents, as in CT scanning. Fig. 5.3 is an example of this technique, showing the distortion of the right posterior cerebral artery by the tumour visible in the right hemisphere of this brain.

Before the advent of MRI, examination of the spinal cord also required the introduction of a contrast agent to the cerebrospinal fluid and subsequent X-ray examination. The MRI images in Fig. 5.8 are direct, and clearly show the cystic tumour with consequent dilation of the cervical spinal cord.

While MRI is often complementary to CT scanning and other radiological and ultrasonic methods, it is important to stress the following unique advantages of the technique:

1. It does not use ionizing radiation.
2. An arbitrary slice of any organ can be imaged.
3. Images of successive slices can be acquired.
4. MRI is able to image pathological processes within the vertebral canal and the skull as well as abnormalities of the cerebrospinal fluid.
5. MRI uses mainly natural sources of contrast between different tissues.
6. MRI can image the vascular system without catheterization or administration of contrast agents.
7. Localized spectroscopy can monitor metabolites in selected regions of tissue.

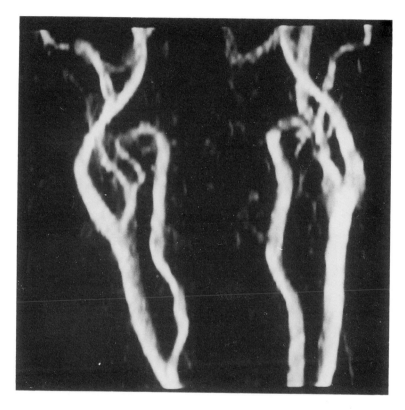

Figure 5.1, MRA TOF. Both carotid trees are shown. The bifurcation of one common carotid is seen. The early part of the internal carotids is normal. The external carotid arteries are also normal, and of normal diameter.

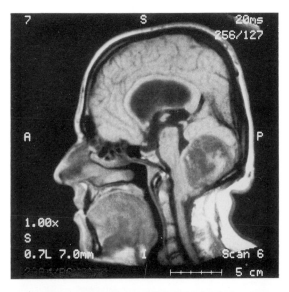

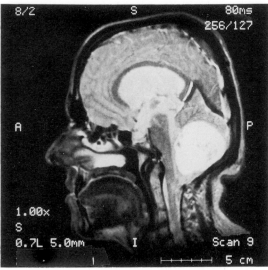

Figure 5.2. Image of the brain in the sagittal plane. **Above:** SE, TR = 600 ms, TE = 20 ms, T_1-weighted image. **Below:** SE, TR = 2000 ms, TE = 80 ms, T_2-weighted image. A large cystic tumour with inhomogeneous MRI signals is visible in the posterior cranial fossa. The mass of the tumour presses on the fourth ventricle. The lateral ventricles and the aqueduct are expanded through restriction of the outflow of cerebrospinal fluid and the intrusion of the tumour into the foramen magnum. The image is consistent with an astroglioma of the cerebellum.

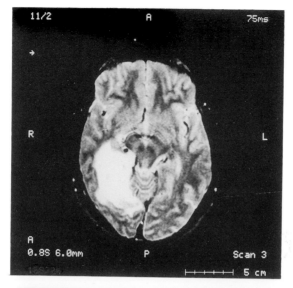

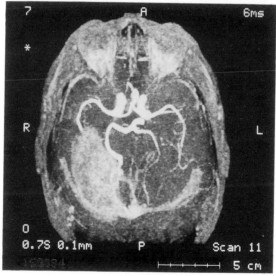

Figure 5.3. Image of the brain in the transaxial (approximately horizontal) plane. **Above:** SE, TR = 2000 ms, TE = 75 ms. An abnormal mass in the parietal lobe of the right hemisphere of the brain and a compressed deformed right cerebral peduncle are visible. **Below:** TOF angiography of the intracranial blood vessels. Reconstruction in the axial plane. The right posterior cerebral artery is distorted anteriorly. There is a network of pathological vessels in the region of the tumour. The image is consistent with a glioma of the right parietal lobe.

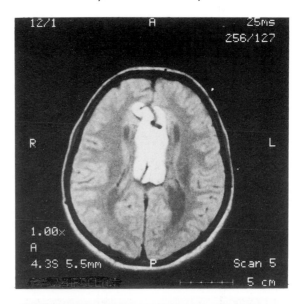

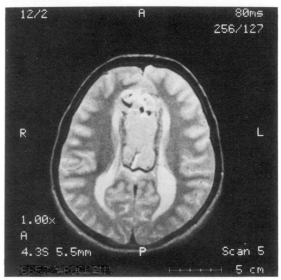

Figure 5.4. Above: SE, TR = 2000 ms, TE = 25 ms, T_2-weighting. **Below:** SE, TR = 2000 ms, TE = 80 ms, T_2-weighting. The abnormal mass within the corpus callosum gives enhanced MRI signals. The lateral ventricles are deformed by the mass of the tumour growing into the third ventricle from above. The image is consistent with a lipoma of the corpus callosum.

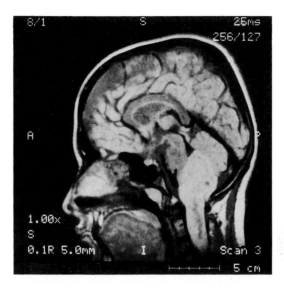

Figure 5.5. SE, TR = 2000 ms, TE = 25 ms. A tumour giving enhanced MRI signals is visible within the cerebellum, the medulla oblongata and the cervical spinal cord to level C4. The tumour fills the foramen magnum.

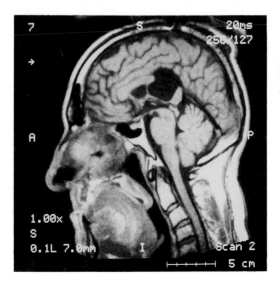

Figure 5.6. SE, TR = 600 ms, TE = 20 ms. Image in the sagittal plane. A congenital defect of the brain. Only the anterior part of the corpus callosum is seen.

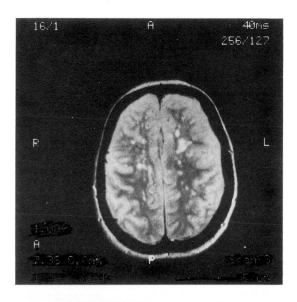

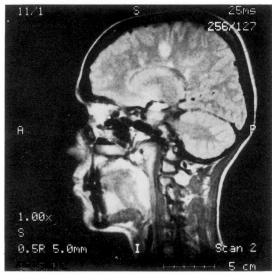

Figure 5.7. Above: SE, TR = 2000 ms, TE = 40 ms. **Below:** SE, TR = 2000 ms, TE = 25 ms. T_2-weighted image of the brain in the axial and sagittal planes. There are foci of variable size giving enhanced MRI signals in the white matter of the brain in the neighbourhood of the lateral ventricles. The changes may be demyelinating.

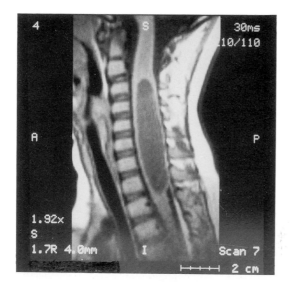

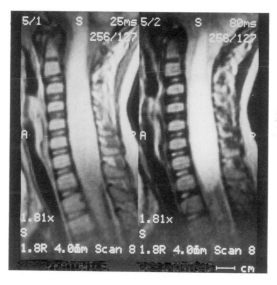

Figure 5.8. SE, **Above:** TR = 600 ms, TE = 30 ms, T_1-weighting. **Below left:** TR = 2000 ms, TE = 25 ms. **Below right:** TE = 80 ms. Image of the cervical spine in the sagittal plane. An abnormal mass is seen within the cervical spinal cord. This is a cystic tumour from C2 to T2 with consequent dilation of the cervical spinal cord, constriction of the sub-arachnoid space and a region of oedema above and below the tumour. The image is consistent with an astroglioma of the spinal cord.

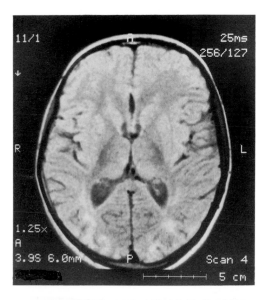

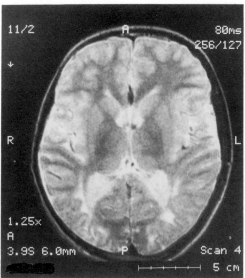

Figure 5.9 SE, **Above:** TR = 2000 ms, TE = 25 ms. **Below:** TR = 2000 ms, TE = 85 ms, T_2-weighted image of the brain in the axial plane. Changes giving increased MRI signals in the cortex and the white matter of the parietal and occipital lobes are seen in both hemispheres of the brain. The lateral ventricles are enlarged. From the MRI examination and additional clinical tests, subacute sclerosing panencephalitis was diagnosed in this patient (an 11-year-old child).

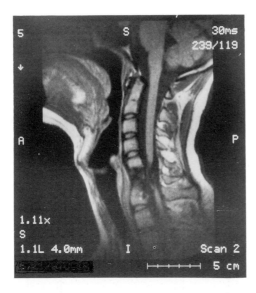

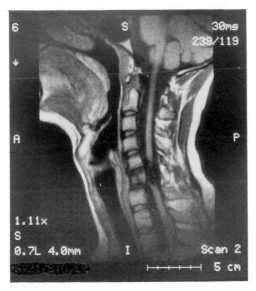

Figure 5.10. SE, two neighbouring slices, both with TR = 600 ms, TE = 30 ms, T_1-weighted images of the cervical spine in the sagittal plane. Fracture of the body of C6 is demonstrated, with displacement towards the vertebral canal and discontinuity of the cervical spinal cord at the C5–C6 level.

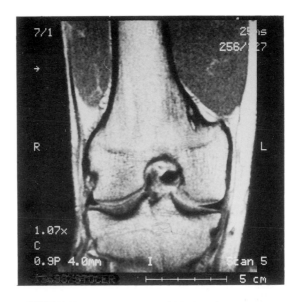

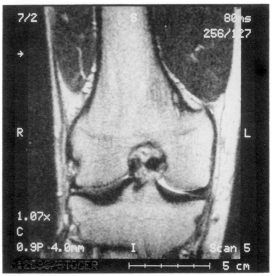

Figure 5.11. SE, TR = 2000 ms. **Above:** TE = 25 ms. **Below:** TE = 80 ms. Images of the right knee in the coronal plane, with collateral menisci and cruciate ligaments normal.

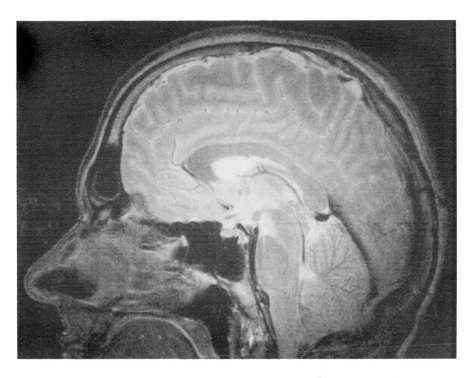

Figure 5.12. T$_2$-weighted image composed of 512 rows and 512 columns obtained using a 3 T Bruker MRI tomograph. Pixel size 0.5 mm × 0.5 mm, slice thickness 3 mm.

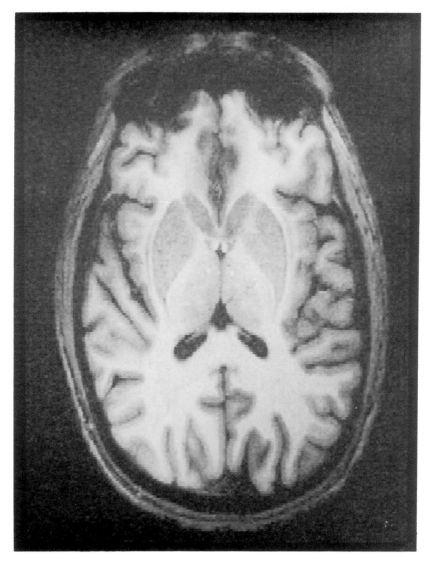

Figure 5.13. T_1-weighted image composed of 256 rows and 256 columns obtained by inversion recovery (IR) using a 3 T Bruker MRI tomograph. TIR = 1 s, TR = 2.5 s. The signal from the cerebrospinal fluid is extinguished.

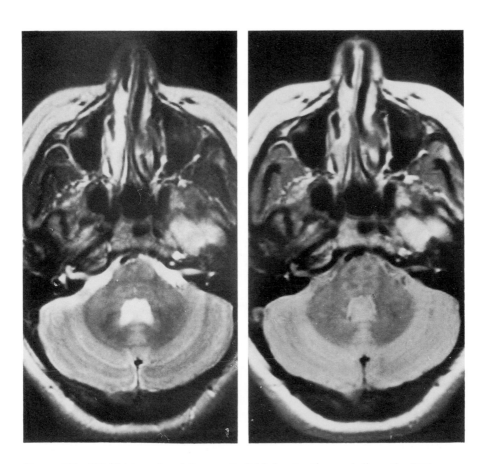

Figure 5.14. MR SE images in a 2 T magnetic field showing the cerebellum, the VIII nerve within the petrous temporal bone (bilaterally), and the maxillary sinuses. The image on the left is proton density-weighted because it was obtained with a short echo time (TE = 20 ms). The right-hand image has mixed weighting (TE = 80 ms). Parameters of both images: TR = 3500 ms, 256 columns, 256 rows. MRI tomograph Gyrex 2T-D1x, made by Elscint, with a 2 T field.

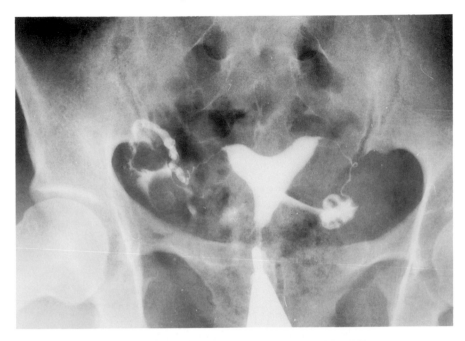

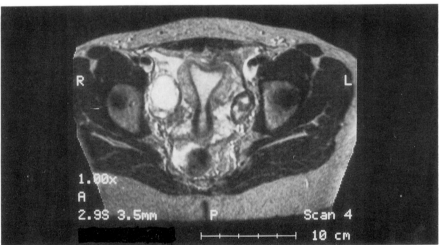

Figure 5.15. Above: X-ray image of a congenital defect of the uterus taken using a contrast agent. **Below:** In the MRI image of the same patient the concave outline of the lower segment of the uterus reveals a bicornuate uterus. The diagnosis was confirmed by laparoscopy. (Figure kindly supplied by Dr. P. Twarkowski.)

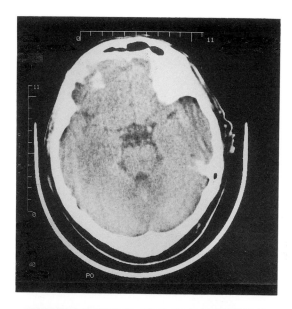

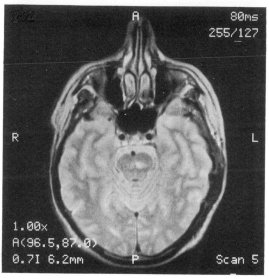

Figure 5.16. Above: CT scan of the brain (using X-rays) shows a small low-density focus at the left of the pons. **Below:** The T_2-weighted MRI image of the brain of the same patient reveals two paravascular foci in the pons, symmetrically located on each side.

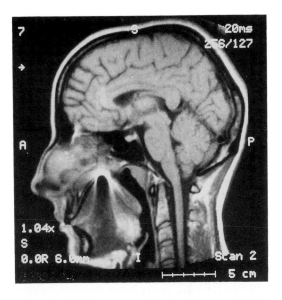

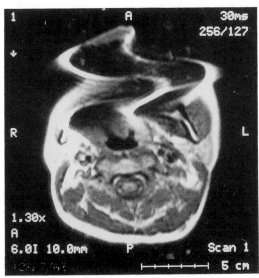

Figure 5.17. Artifacts caused by the presence of magnetic foreign objects in the body. **Above:** T_1-weighted image in the sagittal plane shows interference from a metal dental bridge. **Below:** Image in the transverse plane at the level of the third cervical vertebra. The interference caused by a metal structure in the jaw does not reach the spinal cord.

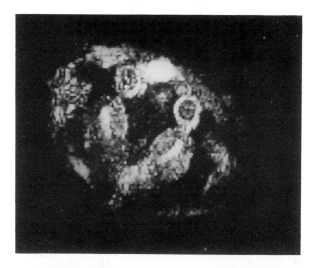

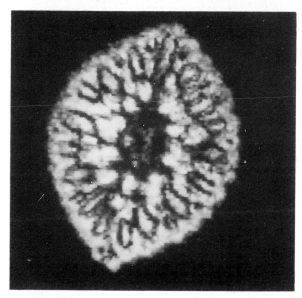

Figure 5.18. MRI microtomography. **Above:** Transverse section through the body of a drone bee showing testicles, spermatic duct and vascular system. Slice thickness 0.4 mm, resolution in the cross-section plane 0.03 mm, magnification 18×. **Below:** Transverse cross-section through a joint of the stem of the grass *Dactylis glomerata* showing the vascular system. Slice thickness 0.4 mm, resolution in the cross-section plane 0.025 mm, magnification 22×. Images obtained at 6.4 T field using a microtomograph built by Prof. A. Jasinski and his colleagues at the Institute of Nuclear Physics in Kraków.

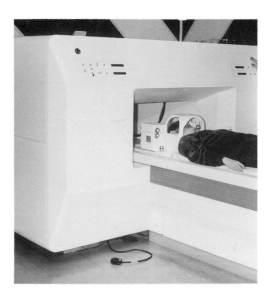

Figure 5.19 Resonex Rx 5000HP MRI tomograph with a 0.5 T electromagnet.

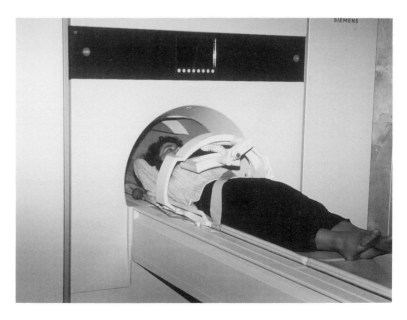

Figure 5.20. Magnetom Impact MRI tomograph with a 1 T superconducting magnet made by Siemens.

5.2 Indications and Contraindications

The general acceptance of MRI as a regular investigation tool relies on the usefulness of the images to the clinician. For example, in the past, treatment of musculoskeletal tumours consisted of amputation of the limb. Since MRI now allows the very precise delineation of such tumours, they can often be excised.

MRI is often successful when there is a clinical indication of a neoplasm, of inflammatory, degenerative demyelinating processes, congenital abnormalities, genetically conditioned diseases of the central nervous system and vascular complaints. Some pathological process occur within anatomical structures inaccessible to examination by other methods. The organs which are imaged best are the lower back part of the skull, the pons, the medula oblongata, the lower part of the pituitary gland and its vicinity and the structures behind the eyeballs. Apart from monitoring pathological changes in the nervous system, MRI is useful for the examination of the mediastinum, neck tissues, the cranium, the vascular and skeletal systems, the breasts and the pelvis. Special MRI programs allow the study of arterial and venous blood vessels, especially when atherosclerotic processes are involved, and of congenital irregularities. Images of joints are helpful to functional studies of human motion.

However, there are situations when the use of MRI is not advisable. Contraindications may be absolute (when the application of MRI is dangerous) and relative (when there is no danger to the patient, but MRI will be ineffective, for example because of significant local distortions of the image).

Absolute contraindications apply with patients using implanted cardiac pacemakers (as magnetic fields may interfere with their operation) and implanted magnetic (ferrous) objects such as artificial heart valves, intracranial metal clips, neurostimulators, metal fragments in the eye-ball, implanted hearing prosthesis in the middle or inner ear or other metallic items in the vicinity of the brain. MRI cannot then be used because of the physical effects of constant magnetic fields on metallic objects and electrical circuits. Cardiac pacemakers may be displaced in the magnetic field, the program may be changed and the action of the pacemaker may become erratic or even cease. It is thus recommended that patients using implanted cardiac pacemakers not only should not be examined by MRI, but should stay away from magnetic fields as weak as 0.0005 T.

Images may be distorted (artifacts) by the presence of the following objects in the patient's body: surgical clamps in the aorta, wire surgical stiches, metal nails used in treating broken bones, artificial metal joints, metal fragments in the body or skin (such as shrapnel fragments), removable dentures, hearing aids, insulin pumps, electrodes of all kinds, intrauterine inserts and other internal metal-containing objects. However, distortions are normally limited to the near neighbourhood of a foreign body and often do not completely invalidate the diagnostic usefulness of the image (see Fig. 5.17). In any case, before carrying out the MRI examination, the operator of the imager should always conduct a detailed interview with the patient in order to establish whether any of these circumstances are relevant.

The effects of the static magnetic field on the human body are unknown. However, it is assumed that, given the sensitivity of fast-dividing foetal cells to a variety of physical influences in the first three months of pregnancy, MRI is not completely safe in the examination of pregnant women.

Apart from the strong constant magnetic field, during an MRI examination the patient is subjected to fast-changing field gradients, the radiofrequency field and the associated "acoustic ringing". A high-frequency alternating field can in principle warm the tissue, but MRI uses fields of small amplitude and thermal effects are thus easily kept within acceptable limits by an appropriate construction of the transmitter-receiver coils. While it must always be used with care by suitably trained personnel, there is no doubt that MRI is considerably safer than other imaging methods, particularly those which use X-rays (CT scanners) or nuclear radiation.

FURTHER READING

*Abragam A., *Principles of Nuclear Magnetism* (Oxford University Press, Oxford, 1983).

Andrew E.R., *Nuclear Magnetic Resonance* (Cambridge University Press, Cambridge, 1969).

Atlas S. W., *Magnetic Resonance Imaging of Brain and Spine* (Raven Press, New York, 1986).

Brant-Zawadzki M. and Norman D., *Magnetic Resonance Imaging of the Central Nervous System* (Raven Press, New York, 1986).

Brown M. A. and Semelka R. C., *MRI: Basic Principles and Applications* (Wiley-Liss, New York, 1995).

*Callaghan P. T., *Principles of Nuclear Magnetic Resonance Microscopy* (Oxford University Press, Oxford, 1991).

Chien D. and Edelman R. R., Ultrafast imaging using gradient echoes. *Magnetic Resonance Quaterly*, **7**, (1991), 31–56.

Edelman R. R., Wielopolski P. and Schmitt F., Echo planar MR imaging. *Radiology*, **192**, (1994), 600–612.

Farrar T. C. and Becker E. D., *Pulse and Fourier Transform NMR* (Academic Press, New York, 1971).

Finn J. P., Goldmann A. and Edelman R. R., Magnetic resonance angiography in the body. *Magnetic Resonance Quarterly*, **8**, (1992), 1–22.

Foster M. A., *Magnetic Resonance in Medicine and Biology* (Pergamon Press, Oxford, 1984).

Foster M. A. and Hutchison J. M. S. (Editors), *Practical NMR Imaging* (IRL Press, Oxford and Washington, D.C., 1987).

Henkelman R. M. and Bronskill M. J., Artifacts in magnetic resonance imaging. *Reviews in Magnetic Resonance Imaging*, **2**, (1987), 1–126.

*Hennel J. W. and Klinowski J., *Fundamentals of Nuclear Magnetic Resonance* (Longman Scientific and Technical, Harlow, 1993).

Higgins C. B., Hedvig H. and Helms C. A., *Magnetic Resonance Imaging of the Body* (Raven Press Ltd., New York, 1992).

Kumar A., Welti D. and Ernst R. R., NMR Fourier zeugmatography. *Journal of Magnetic Resonance*, **18**, (1975), 69-83.

Lauterbur P. C., Image formation by induced local interactions: examples employing nuclear magnetic resonance. *Nature,* **262**, (1973), 190-191.

Lauterbur P. C., Dias M. H. M. and Rudin A. M., Augmentation of tissue water proton spin lattice relaxation rate by *in vivo* addition of paramagnetic ions. *Frontiers Biol. Energetics*, **1**, (1978), 752-759.

Lauterbur P. C., Kramer D. M., House W. V. and Chen C. N., Zeugmatographic high resolution NMR images of chemical inhomogeneity within macroscopic objects. *Journal of the American Chemical Society*, **97**, (1975), 6866-6868.

Mansfield P., Maudsley A. A. and Baines T., Fast scan proton density imaging by NMR. *Journal of Physics E: Scientific Instrumentation*, **9**, (1976), 271-278.

Mezrich R., A perspective on K-space. *Radiology*, **195**, (1995), 297–315.

*Morris P. G., *Nuclear Magnetic Resonance Imaging in Medicine and Biology* (Oxford University Press, Oxford, 1986).

Mugler J. P. III and Brookeman J. R., The optimum data sampling period for maximum signal-to-noise ratio in MR imaging. *Reviews in Magnetic Resonance Imaging*, **3**, (1988), 1–51.

Parker D. L. and Guilberg G., Signal-to-noise efficiency in magnetic resonance imaging. *Medical Physics,* **17**, (1990), 250–256.

Pels R., Tammo H., Davis M. A. and Ros P. B., Intraluminal contrast agents for MR imaging of the abdomen and pelvis. *Journal of Magnetic Resonance Imaging,* **4**, (1994), 291–300.

Rinck P. A., *An Introduction to Magnetic Resonance in Medicine* (Georg Thieme Velag, Stuttgart, 1990).

Shellock F., *Pocket Guide to MR Procedures and Metallic Implants: Update* (Raven Press, New York, 1994).

Schild H. H., *MRI Made Easy* (Schering AG, Berlin, 1990).

Speck U.,*Contast Media. Overview, Use and Pharmaceutical Aspects* (Springer-Verlag, Berlin, 1991).

Wolff S. D. and Balaban R. S., Magnetization transfer imaging: practical aspects and clinical applications. *Radiology,* **192**, (1994), 593–599.

Note: Items marked with an asterisk require the knowledge of advanced mathematics.

INDEX